3 5 7 9 10 8 6 4

Vintage
20 Vauxhall Bridge Road,
London SW1V 2SA

Vintage Classics is part of the Penguin Random House
group of companies whose addresses can be found at
global.penguinrandomhouse.com.

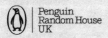

Penguin
Random House
UK

First published in Great Britain in 2010 by Harvill Secker
This short edition published by Vintage in 2017

penguin.co.uk/vintage

A CIP catalogue record for this book is available from the British Library

ISBN 9781784872595

Typeset in 9.5/14.5 pt FreightText Pro
by Jouve (UK), Milton Keynes
Printed and bound by Clays Ltd, St Ives plc

Penguin Random House is committed to a sustainable future for
our business, our readers and our planet. This book is made from
Forest Stewardship Council® certified paper.

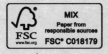

# Calm
## TIM PARKS

VINTAGE MINIS

# Author's Note

How did I come to be where the reader will find me at the
beginning of these pages? Not by careful planning, nor any
deep wish of mine, and certainly not in order to report
back this experience to the world. Quite the contrary. If
there was one thing in my life I never imagined myself
doing, it was a Buddhist meditation retreat. Brought up
in an evangelical household with parents who spoke in
tongues and occasionally performed exorcisms, I had
vowed to spend my life as far as possible from anything
that smacked of spirituality. Then, in midlife, chronic pain
struck. I won't describe the details, but they were embarrassing. Let's say my lower abdomen felt like a lump of
molten lava. There were urinary issues. The doctors let me
down. They filled me with drugs and offered surgery while
admitting they didn't understand what was up. Nothing
worked. Finally, I had the good luck to discover a book
called *A Headache in the Pelvis* by a certain Dr Wise. It
advised a series of breathing exercises, oddly described as

paradoxical relaxation, which proved an immense help but had the unexpected side effect of leading me to understand that I must change my life. Then an old friend who gave shiatsu massages told me, if you want to learn to relax through breathing, you should go to a Vipassana retreat. So after a year's prevaricating, I did.

# The Gong

Vipassana meditation is done sitting cross-legged like a Buddha. Before confirming my booking, I phoned the meditation centre to warn them that I had never been able to sit cross-legged; I wasn't a flexible guy. They reassured me I could always use a chair. Lying down, however, was not permitted. The back must be upright.

I was anxious.

'The position is not the problem,' a man with a haggard, monkish face announced.

On arrival, I was surprised to find people talking. I had assumed the whole retreat took place in silence. Sitting on the front doorstep of the farmhouse, looking out over an Alpine panorama of peaks and stone and misty cloud, a girl in her mid-twenties had been expressing her concern (and mine) about spending ten to twelve hours a day with her butt on a low cushion.

'The position is not the problem,' this gloomy, handsome man repeated. From the way he spoke it appeared that there was a problem, perhaps a very considerable one, just that it wasn't 'the position'.

What then?

Before departing I had looked up 'Vipassana meditation' on the net:

> **Vipassana** *means seeing things as they really are. It is the process of self-purification by self-observation. It is a universal remedy for universal problems.*

'Universal' and 'remedy', I thought, are two words that when put together can only epitomise wishful thinking, unless we are talking about a bullet in the brain. Purification, on the other hand, was a concept I couldn't begin to understand and hence a goal I could hardly desire. As for seeing things as they are, I knew that meditation was done with the eyes closed.

'Vipassana helps you to start feeling your body,' Ruggero, my shiatsu friend, said. Lots of his fellow shiatsu practitioners did it; it enabled them to explore the meridians. He suggested I look on the retreat as a *merely physical therapy*.

What could that mean from a man who didn't believe in the separation of mind and body?

In the early evening we gathered in the meditation room and were invited to take a vow of silence. Seventeen of us. From now on we wouldn't be able to compare notes. Since the centre advertised itself as a lay Buddhist, non-religious organisation, I was surprised by the liturgical solemnity of the language and the moral seriousness of some of the avowals. For the space of our stay: we mustn't speak or communicate in any way; we mustn't kill, or harm any living creature; we mustn't steal or use what was not ours; we mustn't ingest intoxicants or any mind-altering medicines; we mustn't indulge in any sexual activity; we mustn't disturb those around us; we mustn't read or write; we mustn't engage in any other religious or meditative practice; we mustn't leave the grounds; we mustn't wear shoes in the meeting room; we mustn't lie down in the meeting room; we mustn't sit with our feet pointing towards the teacher.

I had no problem with any of this.

There was one positive instruction: we must ask the teacher, a certain Edoardo Parisi, to teach us Vipassana. He was not proselytising. We must seek him out.

Repeating a formula that was read out to us, we asked. We wanted to be taught.

There was then a 'guided meditation'.

The meeting room was a modern wood-and-glass extension built onto the side of the renovated farmhouse, itself perched on the steep slope of the mountain. Outside, rain fell steadily through the darkness. Inside, the only light came from burning logs behind the glass door of a stove and a dim lamp on the floor. The participants, men to one side, women to the other, sat cross-legged on cushions facing the teacher who was slightly raised on a low dais. Just one elderly lady had chosen a chair. Was it vanity, then, made me choose to sit cross-legged? Looking around as we removed our shoes and entered the room, I had simply copied the others. Against the wall there was a stack of cushions, hard and soft. I put two under my butt and pillows each side of my feet to support the knees. My ankles had to be yanked into position.

There was a long silence. The outside of the feet pressing against the mat would be the first to complain, I thought.

'May all beings live in peace,' the meditation began.

'May all beings be free from all attachment and all sorrow.

'May all beings be happy and enlightened.'

'Sadhu Sadhu Sadhu,' the more experienced meditators replied.

I was taken aback by the religious feel of this – the mumbo-jumbo 'sadhu' in particular – but accepted that it was a rigmarole that must be gone through if I was to enjoy the benefits of the days ahead. There was no assent in my mind. The idea that all beings might ever be free from sorrow was impossible and hence it was impossible for me to wish it. I remembered Emil Cioran dismissing utopian ideas that 'do honour to the heart and disqualify the intellect' and simultaneously warned myself that if I had come to pit my 'superior' intelligence against ancient formulas I might as well have stayed at home.

After another long silence we were invited to concentrate on the sensation of the breath crossing the upper lip as it enters and leaves the nostrils. Already the pressure of my left ankle bearing down on my right was painful. Already the straight back I had forced myself to assume was collapsing into a hunch. How could I concentrate on something so nebulous as breath on the lip in this state of discomfort? Lying down, I might have done it. Lying down I had learned to dispel the tension in my body. Thanks to Dr Wise's relaxation exercises. Cross-legged, tension was intensifying rapidly. Everything went rigid.

I wriggled. Perhaps I had got the position of the cushions wrong. They should have been tipped forward a bit.

I tried to adjust them, tried to sit still. This was hard work.

'If thoughts should arise,' the teacher at last intoned, 'don't worry, it doesn't matter, just say to yourself: thoughts, fantasies, not *my* thoughts, not *my* fantasies, and bring your attention gently back to the breath crossing the lip beneath the nose. The in-breath crossing the lip' – pause – 'the out-breath crossing the lip.'

The voice was soft and reassuring and I tried to follow its instructions. At the same time it was now evident that I had made a mistake coming here. I would never sit through an hour in this position. It had definitely been a big mistake not putting a third cushion under my butt, plus something to ease the pressure where my crossed legs touched. 'Not *my* thoughts,' I repeated, disbelieving. When, for a moment, I felt a light breath on my lip, I clutched at it as a man falling into a fiery pit might clutch at a thread. It snapped. The fiery pit was my legs where pins and needles were advancing rapidly. Amid a turmoil of angry reflections, I remembered something I had translated once from a book on pre-Vedic philosophy: 'So as not to be hurt, before coming near the fire, the wise man wraps himself in the meters.' The arcane instruction had impressed, I remembered it, and I had a vague idea it might now be appropriate in some way, but it also sounded like something from Indiana Jones.

'Thoughts, fantasies,' I repeated determinedly and went looking for my breath again. It eluded me.

'If pains should arise,' came the teacher's quiet voice, 'don't worry, it doesn't matter, just say to yourself: aches, pains, not *my* aches, not *my* pains, and bring your attention gently back to the air crossing the lip beneath the nose. The in-breath crossing the lip' – pause – 'the out-breath crossing the lip.'

Saying 'pain, not *my* pain' worked even less than saying 'thoughts, not *my* thoughts'. Whose pain, if not mine? After twenty minutes the pins and needles had crept up from my crushed ankles to my cramped calves. My thighs were simultaneously burning and numb. My curved shoulders were a rigid block. There would be no warm wave of relaxation tonight. Angrily, I hung on. When the hour mercifully ended, I couldn't stand up.

SO WHY DID you come? I demanded of myself in bed. Surely you didn't really believe this experiment would help you stand up straight. Who cared about standing up straight, anyway? Why had I chosen to give the business of posture such symbolic force?

Oddly, it now appeared that there was a gap between my actually being here, in this remote valley, sharing a room with two younger men (one snoring steadily), and some moment in the past when, presumably, I had had my good reasons for signing up to five days of Vipassana meditation.

Had I thought of it as penitence?

No. Since age fifteen I have refused to think of myself as a sinner.

I stayed awake for some time, got up to go to the bathroom, returned, listened to the man snoring, put in my earplugs, turned to the wall.

'You were looking for a showdown with yourself,' I muttered. That was it. A showdown with this tangled self, these tussling selves. You decided that without that showdown the pains would soon be back. Or other pains.

What form would the showdown take? I had no idea. But I had been told that, sitting in silence for days, people do come to a new knowledge of themselves. That was the goal. Knowledge, confrontation. To plumb the source of my tensions and defuse them once and for all. Settle *once and for all* that 'tussle in the mind'.

Of course, I had no more believed I would be successful in this project than a knight setting out to find the Holy Grail supposes he will be the one chosen to recover it. At some deep level, I wasn't even surprised to have spent a miserable hour merely verifying the fact that my hips, legs and thighs were too stiff for me to sit cross-legged. What else had I expected? Yet the following morning, after a tedious night taking care not to wake my room-mates as I padded back and forth to the bathroom, I went once more to the cushions, not to a chair. And I went *without hesitation*. I went cheerfully, *expectantly*.

In the end, I no longer believe that it is given to us to understand why we behave as we do. I should stop trying.

I say 'the following morning'. In fact the gong sounded at four a.m. Dead of night. It was a rather beautiful gong, a sort of auditory moonlight rippling through the deep silence of the house, promising calm and clarity. I was already awake and went downstairs at once. In the kitchen were flasks of herb tea. I poured something minty and went outside to drink it under the eaves of the house looking out into cloud and fog. A woman about my own age came and lit a cigarette beside me. It wasn't unpleasant, standing silently there together, listening to trees and gutter as they dripped, smelling her cigarette smoke in the damp air. I remember she shifted from one foot to the other. The not-talking actually made us more aware of each other's presence.

At four thirty the gong sounded again and the meditation began. Unguided, two hours. Seventeen people breathing, sniffling, coughing. Some wore hoods or swathed head and shoulders in blankets against the chill, which gave the scene a monkish feel. I had built my seat a little higher and brought a T-shirt to fold between my ankles. I did not expect these small expedients would bring comfort, nor did they. After half an hour toes, feet, ankles, knees, thighs and hips welded together in a scorching pyre from which my curved trunk rose like the torso of some broken martyr. Round this carnage, thoughts flitted and circled like bats in smoke. It would be impossible to convey how many thoughts arose, or how ferociously they blocked all attempts to focus on my breath. There had been nothing of comparable intensity when I had begun the paradoxical relaxation at home with Dr Wise. If, for three seconds, I did focus wordlessly on the sensation of breathing, immediately a yell of self-congratulation was raised, followed by a pertinent reflection on the inappropriateness of such a yell, then another reflection, equally pertinent, that this verbalised statement of inappropriateness only compounded the problem, then another reflection that such pertinent reflections were stealing away the experience that I had come for, the experience of wordlessness. Reflection comes at the expense of being, I told myself. Perhaps especially when pertinent. I was pleased that I had framed the idea so succinctly. And ironically. Would I be able to remember these words at the end of the session? How could I make myself remember, without pen and paper? Oh, but what is the point, Tim, of trying to meditate if you are only interested in describing the perversity of everything that prevents you from doing so?

So it went on. A mental seething. A stampede of cows, flies buzzing round shit, rats at a corpse. By some cruel stroke of irony, our farmhouse was situated in a valley with at least three churches whose mixture of clocks chiming the hours and bells summoning the faithful kept one constantly aware of time passing, and thus hopeful of an end, but also constantly confused as to how much time had passed, and thus despairing when no end came. If I opened my eyes and turned a little I could see the watch which the companion to my left had placed on the floor beside him. But what was the sense of checking the time? What was the point of being here if I was merely yearning for the two hours to be over, my mind projected into the future when I was supposed to be savouring the present – 'the present where there is no conflict' the teacher had said in yesterday's guided session? What did that mean? On the other hand, how savour the present when the present was pain, pain that I knew would dissolve the moment I made up my mind to move? But when I did move, swaying my trunk back and forth, for example, or, more radically, uncrossing and re-crossing my legs, then, after a moment's relief, the hot pain returned stronger still. It was worse.

Accepting defeat, I opened my eyes. There was no sign of dawn. The dark windows were a glossy mirror. The fire glowed red. Raised on a low platform, the teacher, in his early sixties, balding, blond, with a fine, pointed nose, sat in perfect stillness, swathed in a thin white blanket. Around me, others too sat perfectly still. One young man in particular had a wonderfully straight back, a marvellously smooth face. The woman to my right sat in a half lotus, unflinching, motionless, her breast rising and falling very slowly and gently. I envied them. And I held on *because* of them. Something about that young man, at once virile and serene, focused and silent, seemed to rebut my sophisticated objections. Closing my eyes again, I struggled once more to find this elusive point where breath and skin met. Perhaps for a whole minute then, I had the impression that the air coming in and out of my nostrils was a silver thread passing through transparent water. All around me was dark still transparent water and this delicate, mercurial thread of air ran gleaming across it connecting me to some distant point beyond my ken.

HAD I LEFT the retreat after lunch on day three, I would never have 'meditated' again. On the evening of the second day two young men disappeared. I heard angry voices from the garden during the afternoon break and at the evening session they were gone. If I had left with them, I could have read a book, or gone running, or canoeing, or for a walk with my wife, Rita, and the dog. Halfway through the third morning, another place was empty. The maestro spoke calmly of 'right effort, right concentration, right awareness'. 'If you experience pleasure in your meditation,' he said, 'do not attach to it with yearning. If you experience pain, do not attach to it with aversion.'

Attachment with aversion was a new idea to me. But I sensed at once what he meant. It was like when I read an author I despised *because* I despised him, because I enjoyed thinking what a scandal it was that this man was a celebrity.

Or when I kept complaining about a colleague at the university because my identity was intensified by my opposition to him. Or when I listened to the radio outside Ruggero's study *in order* to loathe it. Did I attach to pain in the same way? Scratching sores. Was it possible that this grand showdown with myself that I had planned and been denied actually had to do with the pain I was now experiencing? The showdown was taking place without my realising it *was* the showdown. Why else would I continue to sit cross-legged, without a break, when others had chosen to remove to chairs from time to time?

This form of meditation where you concentrate entirely on the breath was called Anapana, we were told, and merely preparatory to Vipassana, which was something quite different and more challenging. Only when the mind had been tamed and tied down to the breath crossing the lip, like a dog to a chain, could we progress. That would be the fourth day. I knew I wouldn't be ready. But on the third evening, towards the end of the last session, something happened. In the midst of the usual fierce pains, with a strange naturalness and inevitability, my consciousness at last fused with my upper lip: the breath, the lip, the mind, these apparently incompatible entities did, in fact, fit together, flow together, were one. I was my lip bathed in soft breath. At once the breathing that had been irregular and forced subsided to a light caress passing back and forth across the skin, a soft rising and falling breathed, not by me it seemed, but by my whole body, by the air outside my body, by everything around me. Then, as if at the touch of a switch, the scalding rigidity tensing thighs and hips dissolved. In a moment, the lower body sank into suppleness. Where there had been formless pain, I became aware of thighs, knees, calves, ankles, feet. A strange heat was being forced downward through them. My bare feet were cold but a hot pain was passing out pleasantly through the soles.

The experience could not have been more unexpected. Or more welcome. I was immediately anxious it must end at once, anxious that some malignant thought would rise up to cancel it out. Don't think, Tim. Do *not* think! Do not give yourself commands not to think! Silence! I focused on that breath that now seemed so strangely detached from me, or rather that I was just a small part of, as if the boundaries that routinely separated me from the world that was not me had blurred. And after perhaps a minute – but there is no measuring time in these circumstances – like a prisoner released from a yoke, my back, which had been cramped and bent, rose gently upright and was straight. As it did so, I was aware of each of the muscles that quietly lifted it. I felt how natural the erect position was. I felt blessed.

A few moments later and things were back to normal: the pain, the frustration, the waiting for the gong that would bring release.

**Don't think, Tim. Do *not* think! Do not give yourself commands not to think! Silence!**

## Surprise Party

ON THE FOURTH DAY, I wept. It is more embarrassing to talk about this than about my urinary troubles, but to miss it out would be to lose a turning point.

I had got through the two-hour early-morning session. There had been no repeat of the previous evening's brief beatitude, but a corner had been turned nevertheless, for I discovered that the more I let go, without worrying when each session would end or what I was thinking or feeling, then the less the pain of sitting like this bothered me. Rather, it was now as if this cross-legged pain were helping me to discover a movement of the mind that I had never really made before: unquestioning acceptance, letting go. It had been hard work getting to this point and it was not until I discovered that movement, or rather until it simply happened to me, that I even appreciated it was possible. Words can describe a mental experience, after the event, but had the same words been spoken to me a thousand times before the experience, I would no more have understood them than a child born in the tropics would understand sleet and snow. That gloomy man had been right: the position was not the problem. The problem was in my head.

So I sat, still in some pain but no longer angry. And the less I was angry the less I was in pain. At times the position began to feel comfortable, even beautiful, the way it invited stillness: the legs locked, the back anchored, the hands quietly joined, and the mind too seemed to have been quietened *by the position*. Everything came from having accepted that one really was here for the whole five days, from truly *not* wishing for the time to hurry by, truly *not* wanting to be back at one's computer writing it all down.

How right they had been to forbid us pens and paper!

After the morning session, at six thirty, we went to breakfast. We picked up plates, queued at a small table stacked with food, then sat together in silence. I had not expected what a pleasure this would be. The long hours spent wrestling, eyes closed, with wayward thoughts seemed to have heightened our sense of taste. Everybody ate slowly and with relish. A piece of fresh white bread seemed as good as any cake. And each face took on a calm and dignity that made one feel unusually happy to be part of the human race. There was no competition for attention, no flirting or coteries, no exhibitionism, no privileged partnerships. In short, nothing for a story. If you needed milk or water or tea, people understood and offered at once, with a faint smile. Afterwards, each person went to the sink and washed his plate and cup. No wonder they called it the Noble Silence.

But this morning I didn't make it to the food. Leaving the meditation room, you stepped into the small garden, whence it was a few yards to the door into the house and the dining room. On the threshold, I felt a sob rising from chest to throat.

The novelty of the experience was that I was not feeling unhappy in any way. Rather the contrary. Also unusual was my immediate appreciation that what was happening was beyond the usual social controls. My body had decided to sob, the way when it's ill, it decides to vomit.

I stepped aside to let the others pass and, to hide my face, turned to look out over the low garden parapet across the broad valley with its shreds of cloud and shafts of sunlight, its villages and churches, and then, beyond the valley, the great chain of mountain peaks: woods, scree, snow.

The weeping burst on me like a storm. I shook.

This crisis lasted half an hour. On two occasions I tried to go in to eat – I was hungry – but each time the emotion surged up with renewed force. My throat ached. So I sat on a stone table under a pergola and continued to gaze through my tears across the valley which seemed intensely part of the experience, as if, again, there were nothing separating self and outside – I was truly *in* this huge panorama, mind and body, weeping.

Then, as though a voice were calling a class register, name after name was announced to my mind, people I knew or had known; and together with the names came faces, bodies, vivid expressions and gestures. One after another, faster and faster, these folk were crowding into consciousness. It was as if, at some carefully engineered surprise party, a door had been thrown open and I was confronted with everyone who ever mattered to me: my wife principally and throughout – we had been together thirty years – then my son, my daughters, my mother and my father, my brother and sister, my friends, lovers, everybody precious, but colleagues too, old acquaintances, neighbours even, they were all here beside me on the terrace under the pergola looking out over the valley, not summoned by myself, not expecting to see me, but glad nevertheless to be here at this impromptu gathering – and solemn too, solemnly aware of our shared mortality, aware that some had already passed on, while others of us were well on our way through life's journey. Then I saw that the long valley we were gazing over *was* the journey. I was one with the group, the living and the dead, and we were one with the landscape. And slowly, between fits of bewildered tears, it dawned on me, at long last, that the roads to health and to death were one: to recover my health, fully, I must accept death as I had accepted the pain sitting cross-legged in the meditation room. I couldn't do that. I just couldn't. But I knew that if I did, this was what they meant by purification.

I have never wept so deeply. Like most people, I have sometimes been very unhappy, and sometimes very happy.

But there had never been this outpouring, nor this feeling simply of being present, a mere witness, while something necessary unfolded. Had I wanted to resist, I could not have done so.

Finally, when it really was over and I could go to the bathroom to wash my face, I was struck, glancing in the mirror, by this obvious thought: that the two selves that had shouted their separateness on waking that morning almost a year ago were my daily life on the one hand and the ambitions that had always taken precedence over that life on the other. I had always made a very sharp distinction between the business of being here in the flesh, and the project of achieving something, becoming someone, writing books, winning prizes, accruing respect. The second had always taken precedence over the first. How else can one ever get anywhere in life? That was why I had been so challenged when Dr Wise warned me that I must put my painful and embarrassing condition at the centre of my 'project'. What he had meant, I saw now, was that the real project was always mortality.

THE NEXT MEDITATION session was not till eight a.m., and, retiring to my bed in the meantime, I called up a thousand bookish references to get a fix on what had just happened to me, to turn it, as always, into words. 'Life presents itself first and foremost as a task. We take no pleasure in it except when we are striving after something.' I remembered reading that, but couldn't remember where.

It had sounded a warning, I had made a mental note. But over the years I had read a hundred warnings and made a thousand mental notes and none had carried the conviction of the ugly bellyache that had stopped me sitting at my computer.

'We go to novels for life.' I had read those words, or words to that effect, quite recently, in James Wood's book *How Fiction Works*. But they might easily have been spoken by D. H. Lawrence or F. R. Leavis. And I understood now with absolute certainty that this claim was a false and self-regarding piety. Life is *not* in novels. The novels that most compellingly keep us away from life are those that most accurately, intensely and wonderfully imagine it and replace it for us, the novels of Dostoevsky and, yes, of Lawrence, of the truly great writers. But the novels themselves are *not* life and we don't go to them for life. If it's life we want, we put the book down. There were some dumb lines from O-level Browning:

> And you, great sculptor – so, you gave
> A score of years to Art, her slave,
> And that's your Venus, whence we turn
> To yonder girl that fords the burn!

'Yonder', 'fords' and 'burn' were awful, I thought. Why had such poor poetry stuck in my head?

Or there was Poe's story about the painter who so obsessively has his young wife sit for her portrait, that only when the absolutely life-like painting is finished does he notice the girl is dead. Art at life's expense.

Then I remembered – the weeping experience had set my brain racing – Robert Walser and the Benjamenta Institute of his novel *Jakob von Gunten*. Yes. Jakob, the narrator, is sent to a school where he must 'learn to think of nothing', something he at first finds absurd, but that eventually wins him over. 'One must go courageously into the inevitable,' was a line I remembered.

But why seek to tie down the intensity of what had happened to me with all these literary references? First the emotion, then the excited reflection on emotion, attempting to divert it from its initial function, to enrol it in my career project, to turn it into smartness and writing. First the illness to warn you away from monomania and back to life and then the reflection on that process, moving you away from life and back to monomania, back to writing and books. Was that what Wordsworth meant by 'Emotion recollected in tranquillity.' The formula sounded so innocuous, but the next logical step was to seek the emotion *in order* to recall it in tranquillity, to care more about the recollection than the emotion, because it was the sophisticated recollection that brought recognition and celebrity and self-esteem. 'Who can ever feel at ease when he cares about the world's praise and admiration?' *Jakob von Gunten* again. I had remembered that line too. More warnings. Jakob comes to appreciate the school's curriculum of thinking about nothing because he is disturbed by the power and ugliness of the instinct to achieve. I remembered an anecdote about Walser. One day his admirer, Carl Seelig, went to visit him in the mental home where he lived. You know, Robert, Seelig told him, you are perhaps the greatest writer in the German language at this time. Walser was upset. If you ever say such a thing again, he told Seelig, I will never speak to you.

I lay on my bed, leafing through the pages of my literary memory. As I did so I knew that it was foolish. The thing to do was to get back to the silence. Go to the meditation room now, I told myself, even *before* the next session. Go and sit in silence. At once a quotation rose to possess even this decision.

> The important thing is not to learn, but to undergo an emotion, and to be in a certain state.

That was Aristotle. I laughed and discovered something that has served me well since: the more we threaten thought and language with silence, or simply seek to demote them in our lives from the ludicrous pedestal on which our culture and background have placed them, then the more fertile, in their need to justify and assert themselves, they become. Reflection is never more exciting than when reflecting on the damage reflection does, language never more seductive than when acknowledging its unreality.

This is the territory of Beckett, I thought. 'Of it goes

on!' *The Unnameable*. The mind's mindless chatter. Beckett too had spoken of being brought to an awareness of his sick psychological state by an array of inexplicable pains.

I stopped myself and went downstairs for the first session of Vipassana.

# *Anicca*

WORDLESS WAKEFULNESS, LIVELY STILLNESS, meditation resists description. When, at the beginning, words and images fizz in resistance to our attempt to put them aside, the writer can have fun. But when thought at last relents, when eyes close behind closed eyes and the mind sinks silent into the flesh, then it's hard to describe that strange state of alertness, oneness, quiet. Moreover, the meditator loses all desire to do so.

To what end?

Vipassana, however, does offer a few fireworks on the way to composure which all practitioners recognise. Something can be told, though the experience lies beyond any verification. Above all, you can't see it. There is nothing you can copy, the way we might all copy the movements of a tennis player, or the way Eugen Herrigel copied his Zen master of archery.

'Now,' our teacher says, 'take your concentration away from the breath crossing the lip, and raise it to the top

When thought at last relents, when eyes close behind closed eyes and the mind sinks silent into the flesh, then it's hard to describe that strange state of alertness, oneness, quiet centre of the head, a small area, about the size of a coin, corresponding, in an infant, to the fontanel. Focus your attention there. Take note of any sensations that arise, without seeking to induce sensations where there are none, without resisting or altering sensations when they occur.'

So, at each of the retreats I have been to, whether of five days or ten, of twenty people or of sixty, on the fourth morning, it begins. Never, at first attempt, do I find any sensation in this neglected area of my anatomy: the bald spot. I can't even locate it. What does happen is that a headache flares as the mind detaches from the breath and moves out to explore the body. The tension swells into the skull for a few seconds, then fades.

Superficially, the Vipassana process is not unlike Dr Wise's paradoxical relaxation. One is to contemplate sensation as it flows and ebbs throughout the body. The difference lies in the intensity and thoroughness of the exploration and the attitude with which it is undertaken. One renounces any objective beyond the contemplation itself. You are not here *in order* to relax, or to overcome pain, or to resolve a health problem – the experience is not subordinated to a higher goal – you are here to be here, side by side with the infinitely nuanced flux of sensation in the body.

First the fontanel, then the forehead, then the temples (left and right), the back of the head, the ears (left and right), the eyes (left and right), the nose, the nostrils (left and right), the cheeks (left and right), the lips (upper and lower), the gums (all), the teeth (every one), the tongue (above and below), the pallet, the jowls (left and right), the throat, the jaw, the neck.

And we have only just begun. The body is a universe. It has many parts. It is made up of many materials. The skin, the muscle, the nerves, the tendons, the blood, the bone . . .

But what does it mean that the mind, or the attention, *moves* around the body? The body is absolutely still (you are not flexing muscles to feel, as you did in the early days of paradoxical relaxation), yet, within the three-dimensional stillness of limbs, head, trunk, you have the impression of the mind shifting, exploring, travelling up and down, left and right, as if, with the body parts that are usually in movement now firmly anchored, the usually anchored mind can move at will. And this is not the movement of the schoolboy's eye over diagrams of anatomy. It is not the movement of looking. Rather it is like a man wandering through the rooms of a house, in the dark, knocking on this door and that, perhaps after a long absence, checking if anyone is home, if anyone wants to talk, or gripe, or rejoice, or simply turn on a light for him.

For a while, perhaps, there will be no response. The doors are closed, perhaps locked. You must be patient. Nobody has passed this way for some time and it would be impolite of you to start rattling the handles. This is not a police raid.

The forehead doesn't respond.

The ears don't respond.

The nape of the neck never responds.

In another part of the house, on a lower floor perhaps, a noisy melodrama demands your attention. A fierce cramp is shouting in the calves. An ache hammers at the back. These people want an argument. They are protesting. But those are not the doors you are knocking on now. Their turn will come. For the moment you tap politely at the nose. You listen politely to the skin at the bridge of the nose.

No response.

But you have time! Hours of time. You are not in a hurry. There are many doors to try.

Attention attends, unrequited.

Then, all at once, the temples!

I remember distinctly, my first session of Vipassana, it was in my temples that it began. First one, then the other: singing, buzzing, dancing. Had I wished to induce a sensation in this part of the body, I would never have imagined such mayhem, as though insect eggs had hatched, or breath on ashes found a nest of live embers. Yet it wasn't creepy. And it wasn't hot. It was the lively sparkle of freshly poured soda water.

In my temples.

At this point you realise that focusing the mind – eyes closed – on a part of the body is quite different from focusing on something outside yourself, a ball, say, or a bottle, or a boat. In that case the object remains an object, however long we look at it. But like light through a lens, or through a glass of still water perhaps, the mind sets the body alight, or the body the mind. It is hard to say which; the skin glows in the mind and the mind fizzes in the skin. Together, neither flesh nor fleshless, or both flesh *and* fleshless, they burn.

This is the beginning of Vipassana.

The inclination now is to enjoy this novel sensation. It's such a relief, after twenty minutes perhaps, to get a response from the body at last, to understand at long last what the teacher was leading you to. So relax now and enjoy. As you relaxed with Dr Wise. This song in the temples, this temple song, is such a pleasurable sensation.

But the teacher is moving on. We must not attach to pleasures as we must not attach to pain.

Nose now.

Lips now.

Tongue now.

The encouraging thing is that once one part of the body has answered your polite enquiry, others too seem more willing to respond: here a band of heat, there a patch of coldness, here a dull throb, now a tingling current. The whole house is waking up and as you pass from door to door each occupant acknowledges your presence by turn-ing something on: now a blue light, now a red, here a coffee grinder, there a TV. The tower block starts to hum.

These varied sensations, our teacher now tells us, are manifestations of *anicca*, which is to say, the constant instability of all things. He invites us to contemplate *anicca*. To know *anicca*, the eternal flux, in our hands, our chests. To recognise that nothing is fixed. Ego, identity, they have no permanence.

Immediately, my thinking mind rebels. My determined self resists. Who needs this mumbo-jumbo – I'm angry – these mystifying foreign words? *Anicca!* Who needs this *theory*? The body may indeed be subject to constant change, but it is also true that it remains largely the same for many years. I recognise my friends year in year out. In childhood photographs, my face is already essentially me, *Tim Parks*.

As I think these thoughts, the temple dance fades, the lights dim, the pain-mongers on the lower floors increase their clamour.

Damn and damn.

I choose to forget the debate and concentrate on sensation. I remember Ruggero: treat it as an entirely physical thing.

The thud of the beating heart, the rise and fall of the diaphragm, a burning hoop around the waist, a warm tremor in the belly – very slowly, part by ageing part, the body was put together. The book I had translated on early Indian philosophy, Roberto Calasso's *Ka*, told the story of the so-called altar of fire. Blessed with longevity, but nevertheless mortal, the lesser gods sought out the first god, Prajapati, whose broken body was dispersed throughout the world, *was* the world, to ask if there was any way they might be 'saved'. 'You must reconstruct my lost wholeness,' Prajapati told them. 'How?' 'Take three hundred and sixty boundary stones and ten thousand eight hundred bricks . . .' The numbers corresponded to the days and hours of the Vedic year. Every brick was an 'intense concentration'.

The altar was built from the outside inward, focusing the mind. Its shape was that of the eagle, bird of eternal wakefulness. If ever you managed to complete the construction, a fire would kindle and the eagle would take flight to the paradise of immortality.

Well, there comes a moment in Vipassana, if you are lucky, if you stay focused, patient, if you learn not to want such a moment, when the entire body links up and ignites. Once, I remember, it began in my wrists. Pulsing waves accelerated into whirling orbits of bright electrons, pure energy, without substance. Contemplating this marvel, it did seem the ego was bleeding away into the hectic flow. If they wanted to call it *anicca*, let them.

But more often, for me at least, it begins when contemplating pain. It is hard to sit with pain in stillness, allowing it to be there, uncomplaining. A knife blade thrust between the vertebrae, for example. But if you do, then, perhaps, just perhaps, for one can never command these things, a sudden intensification will invade the spine, a rush of fierce heat flushes through the chest and dissolves away through arms and legs. The pain is gone. The hunched back straightens, the lungs fill, and the body is one, as if all the doors in a house had been taken away allowing free movement throughout. You are feeling *everything*, simultaneously, or rather, you *are* everything, from toes to fingertips to the hairs on your head. You dance through the rooms, you who never learned to dance.

The first time this happened to me, on the last session of that first retreat, the experience came together with three warm showers. Implausible as science fiction, that small area at the top centre of the head had begun to buzz, to glow, then overflowed in three drenching floods of warmth. A baptism. When the hour ended I jumped to my feet.

IN THE CAR to the station at Maroggia the young man driving was furious. The whole five days had been an utter waste of time. The teacher was a charlatan, a fool. We had been taken for a ride. *Anicca, Anicca, Anicca!* The Buddha was rubbish. Nirvana was rubbish. Reincarnation was rubbish. There is no way anyone can feel the breath crossing his lip. Bullshit. He had been through the pains of hell trying to sit in that dumb cross-legged position when he could have been skiing. He could have been playing tennis.

I believed in nothing, I said, least of all reincarnation, but it had been an important experience for me.

The other man in the car was the gloomy, handsomely haggard fellow who had told us the position was not the problem. Session after session he had sat two places to my left on a cylindrical cushion in granitic stillness. He did not respond to the angry boy who dropped us at the station, but on the train to Milan he told me he ran a very busy car insurance agency. He had been to a dozen such retreats. These were the only days in the year that were truly his own. It was a rule of his, he said, never to speak of his experiences during meditation. However, one aspect of Vipassana still bothered him, indeed had come to bother him more and more, to the point where he was now ready to stop meditating. 'What does it mean,' he asked, 'when they say the thoughts are not *my* thoughts? What can that mean? How can the thoughts not be *my* thoughts?'

# The Booker Speech

No LONGER MUCH interested in standing up straight, I found my back pulling upright by itself. It happened over the spring. Taking my familiar run across the hills, I was surprised to find myself aware of muscles at the base of the spine. How odd. Days later I could feel my shoulders. A slight warm presence. Finally my neck. It was as if skeletal spaces had been very lightly pencilled in. Becoming aware of the muscles turned out to be one with straightening them. Or letting them straighten me. I didn't do anything. I just had to pay attention. The only difficult thing was getting used to seeing the world from a different angle.

'*Complimenti*,' Ruggero grinned. He insisted I looked ten centimetres taller.

No longer interested in prostates, pelvic floors and plumbing problems, I found my pains were gone. Truly gone. I had stopped watching out for them and they had slouched off. The ease and lightness in my stomach and back made walking a pleasure that was at once a powerful sense of nowness and a memory of childhood. I walked very slowly, savouring my body walking. On my way to the café in the morning I nodded at the moustachioed man in the white cowboy hat who had once demanded that I stand up straight. He nodded back, with new respect, I hoped. It became genuinely hard to believe the state I'd been in two years ago. Had it really been *that* painful?

Only the night-time trips to the bathroom remained, three or four. Irreducible to any pathology, they had stayed, I decided, to prevent me from growing too pleased with myself, or to keep the night present.

With varying results, I continued the meditation at home. Paradoxical relaxation was behind me. It had been directly addressed to the symptom and the symptom was gone. I fixed up a mat and a few cushions in a corner of the bedroom and tried to meditate an hour a day. It was at once more comfortable than at the retreat, and less intense. The warm showers did not return. Nor the fierce pains. It was liturgy after revelation.

Knowing that I had scarcely scratched the surface, I signed up to a ten-day retreat in August. This time there would be a famous teacher, an ageing American, John Coleman. I made no attempt to find out about the man or to look up the philosophy that underpinned Vipassana. The last thing I needed was to turn Buddhist. I just wanted the quiet sitting, the increased perception of the body, the Noble Silence. I went confident that there would be no pain this time. I had sorted that out at home. I knew how to sit cross-legged. At times I even experimented with the Burmese position. It's so hard not to feel pleased with oneself.

Since there were sixty participants, the retreat was in an ex-monastery, in the Tuscan hills. Less chic than you would imagine. On arrival, in the fervour of conversation that precedes the vow of silence, all the talk was of Coleman and what a fantastic teacher he was. '*My* teacher,' someone said. '*Il mio maestro.*' 'I switched to Coleman from Goenka,' said another. There was a general rush to place one's mat and cushion towards the front of the meditation room, near the charismatic guru. May all beings be free from all attachment, I remembered, but, not wanting to be left out, I hurried along with them. I got a good place.

Coleman was on his last legs, shuffling, pushing eighty, fat, sometimes fatuous. He spoke slowly in a sonorous voice between heavy sighs, sprawled in a deep armchair, wearing loose jeans and sloppy sweater. A bland smile suggested he too was pleased with himself. Sitting on a table beside him, a young man with only one leg translated his words into Italian in a grating, high-pitched voice. At once this translation business irritated me. It hadn't occurred to me that language would be an issue. Much of the translation was inaccurate and all of it expressionless. There were occasions when it was hard not to shout out better solutions.

Coleman talked about the three refuges, the four truths, the five precepts, the seven stages of purification, the eightfold path to enlightenment, the ten perfections, the Buddha, the Dhamma, the Sangha, karma, anicca, anatta, samsara, dukkha, suffering, the root of all suffering, the remedy for all suffering, the bodhi tree.

What drivel this was, I thought. And why do all faiths – because this clearly wasn't science – share this mad appetite for numeration? The Trinity, the seven sacraments, the ten commandments. It wasn't *worth* translating properly. On the other hand, I always tell my students that translating accurately is a pleasure *in itself* regardless of the inanity of the original. Certainly I was suffering more for the poor translation than the mystical content.

Every few minutes the man behind me – and he was very close behind me – sniffed three times in rapid succession, then cleared his throat, then coughed. To my dismay, when the meditation proper began, fat old Coleman had someone fetch a large kitchen clock and place it at his feet. It was the kind of clock I could have heard ticking about ten miles away. Immediately I thought of all the guestrooms, classrooms, university offices and rented apartments, where the first thing I'd done on arrival was remove the battery from a ticking clock. What a satisfaction that is, killing the sound that constantly returns you to the passing moment, that stops you being elsewhere in your head. Here I was helpless. This will be hell, I decided.

And I hadn't conquered the pain at all. Twenty minutes into the first session I was in agony.

Nor had I learned to sit up straight. My back collapsed, doubled even. My nose was at my feet (my aching feet).

Why? This was *worse* than Maroggia. I should never have come.

The meditation room was narrow and very long and I was about four rows from the front in ripple and cross-ripple of fidgeting and buttock shifting. Every time I thought I might at last be getting a hold on my breathing, every time the pain began to ease up as the mind focused on the skin of the lip, from behind, came, Sniff, sniff, sniff, er er hemmmm! At once the clock ticked more loudly. Sniff, sniff, sniff, er er *hemmmm*! Tick tick TOCK **TOCK**! The volcano that was my haunches threatened to erupt.

'If there are feelings of pain,' the would-be hypnotic Coleman crooned for the nth time, 'just make an objective note, pain pain . . .'

So what would a subjective note be, Mr Coleman? Or a note that was neither subjective nor objective, for that matter? Why pretend there is anything *reasonable* about all this?

For the nth time the one-legged man on the table translated – *fare una nota obiettiva* (does anyone say, '*fare una nota*?') – his voice as bored and mechanical as Coleman's was sonorous and rhythmic.

I now felt homicidal.

From the corridor came the din of someone wheeling a trolley full of plates and cutlery along the monastery's uneven, unending, stone-flagged corridor. First you heard it approach for a minute or more. At the crescendo, it stopped, right outside the meditation-room door. Now I was waiting for it to start again. Was it going to go away or wasn't it? It was teasing us. I couldn't meditate until it moved off, or until I knew it was staying. Then just when you thought it was staying, off it went with a long-drawn-out squeal followed by a great clatter of plates, knives, spoons and pans, like a goods train at dead of night, the rattle, bang and boom sustained for another minute and more before the din began to fade at what I judged must be the turn of the corridor. How many clock ticks before it is gone completely, I wondered? Twenty? I counted. Tick tock. Tick tock. No, ten ticks more. Still the clatter echoed faintly off the stone surfaces. And the rattle. Fainter and fainter, but still faintly there. Tick . . . tick . . . tick. The guy was *deliberately* going slowly! And a jingle of teaspoons. Tick tick tick. Still ever so faintly. Perhaps he was taking a step back for every two steps forward. He was *deliberately* choosing the uneven flagstones, he was rattling the cutlery trays!

Gone, it was suddenly gone. But now the clock's ticking had got into my skin and was stitching my lips together, each tick was a stitch, up and down, through my lips. How could I feel my breath with a needle sewing up my lips? I imagined the first major massacre at a meditation retreat. 'The assailant was a man in his fifties known to be searching for inner peace. It is not clear why he came to the monastery armed with a Kalashnikov.'

At the same time I recognised this package of feelings all too well. This is me, I thought, me of old. Unredeemed TP. Old resentments, dramatisations, would-be black comedy.

You are getting off on being angry now. You're enjoying it, imagining yourself *imaginatively* angry. À la Geoff Dyer who himself wanted to be à la D. H. Lawrence. Gritting my teeth, I hung on to the end of the session and stumbled over a fizz of pins and needles to collapse on the lawn in the garden.

The monastery was supposedly in a secluded area, high on a steep hot hill and surrounded by an impressive stone wall, but the village immediately beneath the hill had arranged its summer fête for this week. At eight in the evening rock music began, as poorly played as Coleman's meditations were poorly translated. The summer air filtered out most of the treble leaving only a dull beat of drum and bass and the lament of a direly strained voice.

Added to which the Olympics were now under way. From the windows of the convent located directly across the courtyard from our meditation room came the sound of nuns cheering on Italian athletes. In China. If there is one thing I loathe it's the Olympic Games, festival of empty pieties, crass patriotism and sophisticated performance drugs. It was extraordinary how excited and patriotic those old nuns were. Apparently it did not occur to them they might be disturbing us. What a terrible, terrible farce all this was. Ten days of my precious and very busy life wasted!

Still I hung on. I had no idea why. My diligence was a mystery to me. One day I wondered if they had deliberately arranged for us to be assailed by these noises to test our meditative stamina.

The routine at these retreats is that you eat breakfast at

six thirty, after the wonderfully quiet early session, lunch at eleven, then just a piece of fruit late afternoon and nothing till the following morning. 'A little hunger in the evening will do no harm,' fat Coleman smiled. The food, all strictly vegetarian, was not as good as the homemade fare at the smaller retreat in Maroggia. Brought in from outside, the pimply caterers grinned at us as if we were picturesque eccentrics. They seemed to take special pleasure in banging down the knives and forks when they laid the table and then shaking them vigorously in their metal trays when they collected them again, as if panning for gold. The fruit in the evening was chiefly kiwis. I'm not fond of kiwis. How can you peel a kiwi without getting sticky fingers? Fifty people queued around two kettles for tea. I had the distinct impression that old Coleman was enjoying little natters with the prettiest woman on the course. I had caught them three times at the turn of the staircase. Talking.

Where was the Noble Silence?

Every other afternoon, for an hour, there was a so-called 'check-up'. In alphabetical order people were invited, four by four, to bring their cushions to the front, sit before the teacher and report on their progress. On the second day, almost everyone spoke of their pain with the sitting position, their difficulty eliminating their thoughts; many complained of a film playing out before their closed eyes, some old drama rehearsed a thousand times with no solution, as when a ghost appears again and again in the same place in the same clothes – an ex-husband, a dead sister – makes the same gestures and is gone, then back. Never there, never not there.

'I'm in a loop,' one man said. He found it distressing.

'I have a big decision to take when I get home, I just can't get it out of my mind, I see the conversation over and over.'

People couldn't identify the place on their lips where breath met skin. When they did identify it, they couldn't focus their attention there, they lost it. 'It must be my moustache,' one man thought. He would shave it. Perhaps they felt the breath going out, but not the breath coming in. Or they could feel it in their nose, but not on their lip. Why was it so important to feel the breath on the upper lip?

'I have a pain in my shoulder, from an accident a few years ago.'

'I keep getting this fierce headache right behind my eyes, it won't go away.'

'My feet are on fire.'

'I've got period cramps.'

To all these people, sitting cross-legged on their cushions before him, Coleman, enthroned in his armchair, gave the same advice. 'You must say, doesn't matter, pain, pain, not *my* pain. You must say thoughts, thoughts, doesn't matter, not *my* thoughts.'

He smiled and settled his bulk.

I felt rage.

Given my place in the alphabet, I knew I wouldn't be

invited to present myself to the grand old man until the third day. Try as I might to eliminate the mental chatter from my mind, I began to go over and over what I planned to say. I would mention my surprise that while I had no problem meditating at home, here I was experiencing all kinds of pains. Why? I sat up straight at home, here my back collapsed. Did he have any advice beyond, pain, pain, not *my* pain?

I thought of all kinds of attractive ways of phrasing this little speech, ways that would make it clear that I was neither an absolute beginner nor a practised meditator. I would say something different from the others. And of course I would speak in English, rather than going through the translator, the lousy translator. Perhaps I could take the opportunity to offer my own translation services.

Then I was angry with myself. What was this, a theatre? A TV show? I remembered how, on being told I was on the Booker Prize shortlist, I had been unable to stop a modest acceptance speech from playing itself over and over in my mind for weeks before the event. Literally for weeks this acceptance speech had driven me crazy. From the moment of the phone call telling me I was on the list to the moment of the announcement that someone else had won, my acceptance speech refused to stop accepting the prize in my head. Each time with some tiny addition, some precious new flourish. The experience was simultaneously infuriating and immensely gratifying. It really was such a clever, ironic, modest speech. People would not be impressed immediately, I thought. They would just think what a nice ordinary guy I was. Only later would they see what a clever speech it had been. Then they would think me doubly clever, and doubly modest for not having wished to impose my full cleverness on them immediately, but with delayed effect, like those fertiliser sticks you put in the ground that dissolve slowly for months.

On and on this speech performed itself for me, on and on and on. And now I was doing the same thing *for Coleman*. At every new pain and ache and itch that arose, every sound that irritated and interrupted, I revised my little speech. I polished my speech, shortened my speech, lengthened my speech. Which was insane. At least for the Booker there was an audience. Would have been an audience. TV! If I'd won. Here there were just sixty people living in silence, trying in silence to achieve some better relationship with themselves, with existence. *What could it possibly matter how I came across to them?* They didn't care about me. I didn't care about them. And then, how can it *ever* truly matter how one comes across? What on earth could anyone care about a Booker acceptance speech? For Christ's sake! And then, I had known from the beginning that I couldn't win the Booker with the novel I had written. My chances were not six to one but six million to one. It was a miracle they had put me on the list with such an angry book that had sentences more than two pages long. They'd never let it win. So preparing my acceptance speech was doubly ridiculous. At least here I was bound to get a hearing. From sixty people. The speech would happen.

Or maybe not. Because now it occurred to me that what I must do was ask to be excused from saying anything. That was the solution. Then I could stop playing the speech over and over in my mind. I might simply announce: 'Please, Mr Coleman, I would rather say nothing.' Or, 'Teacher, I wish to take refuge in the Noble Silence.' That was good. Then people would know that I *did not want* to draw attention to myself. Perhaps I would speak in Italian, so they weren't obliged to marvel at my being English. Except there was my accent, of course. There is always something that gives you away. Then they would be obliged to marvel how well I spoke Italian. Despite the slight accent. And of course I would immediately translate what I had said into English so that Coleman wouldn't have to hear my carefully chosen words from this incompetent one-legged wonder who disturbed us all from time to time by dragging himself in and out of the room on his crutches. Presumably to go to the bathroom.

'I would rather say nothing, if that's allowed,' I would say, in Italian. Or even better, I could approach Coleman in the corridor before tomorrow and, murmuring softly, ask if he could avoid calling me out to the front. Certainly people could hardly say I was looking for attention if I stayed sitting when the others went up to talk.

Or could they?

It was simply maddening how insistently this

meaningless chatter ground away in my head those first three days of the retreat. Perhaps I should confess, I thought, when I was called out to the front, that I had wasted hours and hours of this precious meditation time with self-regarding thoughts about what I should say when called out to the front, thoughts entirely directed to the effect of my performance on the audience rather than an honest comment on the way my meditation was going. Badly, needless to say. Should I be confessional? Or would that have even more *effect*?

Of course I then imagined *writing* about this meaningless chatter and how brilliantly I could deconstruct myself, or someone like me (very like me), in a novel perhaps. I could very cleverly show how useless I was. Should I write a novel or should I make it non-fiction? Which would seem more *necessary*? And if I wrote non-fiction, should I perhaps use a third person, as Coetzee had in *Boyhood* and *Youth*, or accept the slithery candour of the first person like everyone else? Those are strange books that Coetzee wrote. They make you feel uneasy.

It went on and on. I hated it. I couldn't find a way out. After the first retreat I had read Coetzee's essay on Robert Walser and been astonished by a curious fact and by Coetzee's response to it, a fact that now came back to my mind as being extremely pertinent to this speech madness. In his mid-thirties Walser suddenly found that he could no longer hold a pen. His hand became painfully cramped every time he picked one up. He couldn't write. But of course he had to write, otherwise who was he, where were his old ambitions? So he fell to writing with a pencil. And his handwriting changed drastically. Instead of the generously rounded calligraphy of the well-educated young man from the provinces, he now wrote in a script so minuscule that to the naked eye it looked like some indecipherable code. Even experts, Coetzee remarked, cannot be sure they have got it right.

Why could Walser work with a pencil but not a pen? I wondered now, partly as an antidote to playing this idiotic speech over and over in my head and partly because I suspected that, however self-aggrandising it might seem, Walser's problem and my own were not unrelated. And why, in particular, did he talk about his 'pencil method'? Here comes Coetzee's bizarre interpretation. Like an artist using charcoal, the Nobel winner claimed, Walser needed 'to get a steady rhythmic hand movement going before he could slip into the frame of mind in which reverie, composition, and the flow of the writing tool became the same thing'. That is, he needed the rhythmic movement of the pencil to overcome some obstacle which Coetzee wasn't eager to identify.

But why is a pencil more rhythmic than a pen? Is the charcoal analogy pertinent? Painters do not try to execute miniatures in charcoal, do they? Surely if Walser's script had now shrunk to the indecipherably microscopic, the hand movements would have been *more cramped* and not free and rhythmic at all. Isn't it more likely that Walser's problem lay with the egotism and exhibitionism inherent in writing and publication? That was what was cramping his hand. 'Writers do not know what they lost when they sacrificed anonymity,' Walser had written somewhere. Words to that effect. His novels were all glaringly autobiographical, with an alter ego at the centre of each story. Was it possible that the switch to pencil, which, unlike ink, can be erased, gave him a feeling that what he was doing was provisional, could be reversed? And that writing in such a tiny script he was in a way *hiding* his work from others? He was doing it and not doing it. For a while Walser would copy out his pencil manuscripts in a fair hand for the publishers, using a pen. Detached from the moment of creation, or self-revelation, self-affirmation, the pen was mysteriously useable again. But later he left his work in pencil without trying to publish it, and later still he *stopped writing altogether*.

I kept thinking about Walser in relation to this conundrum of self-presentation, of simultaneously wanting to take the stage and truly not wanting to take it, above all not wanting to want to take it, or not wanting to be seen to want to take it. And wasn't there something of the same conundrum in Coetzee's disquieting decision to write his autobiography in the third person? As if he wasn't writing about himself, but someone else. And no one is harder on that someone else than Coetzee in *Boyhood* and *Youth*, that person responsible for his committing the unforgivable indiscretion of writing these books. He was hard on himself because he was writing books about himself. And everyone knew it. Even though he pretended it wasn't himself. That was what he hated. Writing about himself, he wrote against himself. Himself being a writer writing himself. 'Not I,' Beckett proclaimed. Or had a mouth proclaim. A mouth without a face. Without an I, without an eye. 'Shall I never be able to lie upon any subject other than myself?' wonders Malone, or Beckett, in *Malone Dies*. A rhetorical question. No. Pain, pain, not *my* pain. Please. And when Deirdre Bair went to interview Beckett for the biography the first thing he said was, 'So you've come to demonstrate that it was all, after all, autobiographical.'

And it was!

And I was in deep trouble. I couldn't go on. For long periods, as the hours ticked by, I felt I was swaying from side to side and must sooner or later crash to the floor. I began to look forward to it. Or fall on my nose. I was so hunched. It would be such a relief when I crashed on my nose and everyone would see how much I was suffering and then I could stop and take a rest, take a walk, go to bed, go home perhaps. There was now a stabbing pain right between the shoulders. It was ferocious. Stab, stab, stab. Bizarre lights and burning heat radiated out from it. How could I be in so much pain when I knew there was nothing at all wrong with me? What was I learning from all this, I wondered? Nothing. Nothing except that *every single thought* that rose to my mind was in some way *self-regarding*. No, in *every* way self-regarding. Every thought. My analysis of Walser's problem was no doubt accurate, I complimented myself, and fitted in with many other elements in Walser's biography. My sense that Coetzee actually needed to miss the point was in line with his own obvious conflict when it came to presenting himself. But what is there to present, in writing, if not oneself? Even if I wrote about the man on the moon it would be self-presentation. *Especially* if I wrote about the man on the moon. What I must say when I am finally called to the front, I decided, is that these three days of meditation have revealed to me that every thought I think is, in one way or another, an ugly, fatuous form of self-congratulation. Even what appears to be the most searing self-criticism is in fact self-congratulation. A man capable of seeing his worst side, you congratulate yourself. Coetzee is pleased to have been so hard on himself. Nice observation, Tim. Was there no way out of this? How could I stop it, really stop it, *forever*? Without blowing my brains out.

'Gently return your attention to the breath crossing the point on the upper lip. The in-breath crossing the point, the out-breath crossing the point. Nama and Rupa, mind and material. Everything in the world, mind and material. Without identity.'

Tom Pax was called to the front with three other names.

So much for identity. The translator was misreading from his list of names. Pax I'm used to, but I hate it when I'm called Tom.

Knowing that Coleman always proceeded from left to right, I put down my cushion on the far right.

The first man admitted to panic attacks.

Coleman was silent. 'Just concentrate on the breath,' he told him eventually. 'And make an objective note of the fear.'

The second man confessed he kept falling asleep then waking himself up as his body slipped and slumped.

Like the disciples at Gethsemane, I thought, and thinking this was simultaneous with congratulating myself for the pertinent allusion, then wearily ticking myself off for another manifestation of self-regard.

'One does tend to get sleepy the first three days,' Coleman told him. 'It will stop as we go on. Don't be angry with yourself. Make an objective mental note – sleepiness – then return your concentration to the breath on your lips.'

In a late change of plan I decided I would simply say I was having a lot of pain and was finding it hard to concentrate. Nothing else. The most bland summary of what everyone else had said. I hoped that wouldn't sound provocative. I hoped it wouldn't sound anything at all.

I would say it in Italian. Speak in Italian, as if you were one of them.

What was the 'as if' about?

Then the third man confessed that his main difficulty these last two days had been that he had kept thinking about what he would say, now, when he was called to the front. And Coleman laughed. Coleman laughed deep in his fat belly, a really hearty, rumbly, fat laugh, and said he had been wondering when somebody was going to own up to that. He was evidently much amused.

We had been set up.

'And now I'm saying something completely different from what I planned to say,' my companion lamented.

Coleman smiled. 'So you lost the present for a future moment that didn't even happen.'

That was my Booker story exactly.

'We never say what we plan to say, do we?' Coleman added kindly. 'So why not just leave the words till the moment itself? Nothing is at stake here. You're not being interviewed for a job.'

My turn next. Stay to plan, I decided. The new plan, that is. There is nothing worse than the penalty taker who decides at the last second to go for the other corner.

The fat man turned to me. There was a charisma about him. There was a merriment in his heavy features. Sunk in the flesh, the eyes were bright and young.

'Well, Tom Pax?'

I opened my mouth and nothing came out. It's an experience I've had a thousand times in dreams, but never till now in life. I was voiceless. I was supposed to speak and I couldn't say a word. Three or four times I tried. Nothing but air and pain in my throat.

Shaking his head, Coleman looked down on me from his armchair throne with a mixture of condescension and sympathy.

'I don't know what's happening,' I finally croaked. The words were barely audible.

He leaned slightly towards me. 'Why don't you go back to your place?' he said.

## Personally Of Course I Regret Everything

OVER THE NEXT four days I decided I must stop writing. I had just gathered some concentration, tuned my mind to the breathing, allowed the ticking clock to enter my unresisting pulse, to run across my cheeks and lips and up and down my arms, dissolve in my chest and belly, just got myself settled, in short, into the sitting position, into the meditation room, into the company of my fellow meditators, when the time came to switch from Anapana to Vipassana, from breathing to exploration. Then it was like stepping from a darkened bedroom into a burning house. Or coming out of anaesthetic after surgery. First a prolonged explosion deep in the skull, then, one after another, in the dark landscape behind closed eyes, not so much fires as burning rocks, great boulders of obstruction and pain.

After the first hour of this I hurried outside into the afternoon sunshine, overwhelmed by déjà vu. Had I been writing these experiences as a novel, I thought, then the crisis on the mountain terrace that rainy dawn in Maroggia would have been the obvious place for the story to end, with a life-changing breakthrough. But it had not been life-changing. Here I was five months later, back at square one, back with my old self, back with a sense of something that would never budge, with a body that seemed to resist me, didn't want my company.

Back with my bent back.

I watched the others bringing tea and kiwis out into the garden. On day one, day two, day three, people had walked vigorously up and down, or lain on the grass to do sit-ups and stretching exercises. It was a flat, symmetrical renaissance-style garden, a lawn split by a cross of paths. Now on day four everybody was moving in slow motion. People would take a few steps then stop, standing absolutely motionless for five minutes, even ten, transfixed. They sipped their tea slowly, peeled their kiwis as if it didn't matter whether they ever actually ate the fruit or not. Nobody was exercising. I too had lost any desire to exercise. And I had the impression that I wasn't the only one to have been caught out by the Vipassana. There was a shell-shocked look to the young man passing back and forth in front of me, placing one foot in front of another, heel to toe, as if walking a tightrope over an abyss.

Then it seemed to me that the only way to force an irreversible change in my life would be to dump the project that had been driving me, goading me, making me ill, I decided, for as long as I could remember: the WORD

*PROJECT.* If illness is a sign of election in an author, I thought – where had I read that? – then renouncing writing might be a necessary step to being well. Not that I was actually *ill* any more. But I certainly wasn't *healed* either. Otherwise, what was I doing in this crazy place?

Pulling my ankles into place for the next cross-legged hour, I remembered it had been V. S. Naipaul who had said that to me. We were eating lunch together at a conference many years ago. 'A writer must undergo a serious illness,' Naipaul had confided solemnly. This was some years before his Nobel. 'To awaken his conscience.' Which of course was only Naipaul's way of saying that *he* had undergone a serious illness and *he* was one of the elect. The man was nothing if not vain. How could I have fallen for such nonsense? Because he had indeed written some great novels, of course. Then I recalled that moment in *The Information* when one literary author wonders why a rival literary author bothers to keep on writing. And you know at once that the question is really Amis's question. He calculates the man's earnings. Less per hour than a taxi driver makes. Why does he do it? *To avoid facing up to naked, unmitigated, unmediated reality*, the author (and no doubt Amis) decides. Perhaps it was time, then, for me to face up to that: the simply being here, instead of taking refuge in writing about being here. I must go speechless. The moment of aphony at the check-up had shown me the way.

Guru Coleman, I felt, was trying to tell us something similar in his evening talks. The most immediate reality, the *only* reality to which we had access at every moment of our lives, the fat man said, was the breath, this breath, this instant, crossing our upper lip as it went in and out of our lungs. *The* breath, not *our* breath. Everything else was empty imagining.

These evening talks – from six p.m. to seven – were remarkable for their combination of blandness and pessimism. Sprawled in his chair, vapid smile on slack cheeks, ham hands on chubby knees, Coleman lurched into the sort of wet, preacherly parables my father would not have stooped to with a Sunday School class. 'So you want to have a red Ferrari?' Coleman almost crooned to the Italian crowd. He paused at every rest point. 'All your life you have dreamed of a red Ferrari' – pause – 'you *have* to have that red Ferrari' – pause, smile – 'and when you get it?' – pause, deep sigh – 'When you *get* it?'

He didn't bother to say, what then?

Please, I thought, while the translator trundled through his deadpan approximation for the benefit of the very few Italians who hadn't already grasped the idea, please, do me the favour of finding an object of desire that it would be genuinely hard to relinquish.

I must have a certain woman.

I must win the Nobel Prize.

It irritated me immensely that he drivelled on about this red Ferrari. People on meditation retreats are hardly of a kind to sell their souls for a sports car.

I supposed.

Sometimes Coleman felt too tired to talk and had his translator read us something directly in Italian, while he looked on with the same bland smile on his face.

'There are ten levels of awareness in Vipassana meditation,' the translator read swinging his one leg from the table top.

*Sammasana*, theoretical recognition of *Anicca*, *Dukkha* and *Anatta* (change, dissatisfaction, emptiness), through observation and analysis;

*Udayabbaya*, awareness of the appearance and dissolution of *Nama* and *Rupa*, mind and material, through observation and analysis;

*Bangha*, awareness of the rapid change of *Nama* and *Rupa*, like a swift current or a flow of energy; intense awareness of things dissolving;

*Bhaya*, awareness that this existence is terrible;

*Adinava*, awareness that this existence is full of misery;

*Nibbida*, awareness that this existence is disgusting;

*Muncitukamyata*, awareness of the urgent need and desire to flee this existence;

*Patisankha*, awareness that the time has come to work for complete liberation, through *Anicca*;

*Sankarupekkha*, awareness that the time has come to detach ourselves from all contingent phenomena (*sankhara*) and to break with our ego-centred lives;

*Anuloma*, awareness that speeds up our attempt to achieve liberation.

When he reached *Adinava* I began to smile and by *Munci*-whatever-it-was I was laughing. I couldn't help it. It was so *Beckett*, so like Arsene's great speech in *Watt* that I always use with my second-year students, and that always sets me chuckling:

> Personally of course I regret everything. Not a word, not a deed, not a thought, not a need, not a grief, not a joy, not a girl, not a boy, not a doubt, not a trust, not a scorn, not a lust, not a hope, not a fear, not a smile, not a tear, not a name, not a face, no time, no place, that I do not regret, exceedingly. An ordure from beginning to end.

And it goes on:

> The Tuesday scowls, the Wednesday growls, the Thursday curses, the Friday howls, the Saturday snores, the Sunday yawns, the Monday mourns, the Monday morns. The whacks, the moans, the cracks, the groans, the welts, the squeaks, the belts, the shrieks, the pricks, the prayers, the kicks, the tears, the skelps, and the yelps . . .

But why did these lines of Beckett make me laugh, I wondered, the way I was laughing now at *Bhaya, Adinava, Nibbida* – this existence terrible, this existence full of misery, this existence disgusting? Because they were so over the top, I suppose, because the trite rhythms and rhymes showed how misleading language can be, making everything sound hunky-dory while in fact what we were talking about was deep despair, as if I'd recounted my own months of pain as a nursery rhyme.

But it was more than that. I had been laughing at Beckett, I realised, ever since I was an adolescent, because these ideas were *forbidden*. My Anglican parents would never have countenanced such a vision of life. The blandness of the Anglican sermon always ended in optimism: the risen Christ, redemption, renewed commitment, the promise of glory. All my life I had associated blandness with Christian conformity, socialist optimism, complacency; and hence, vice versa, pessimism with non-conformity, intellectual acuity, liberation from coercive fairy tale into unpleasant truth.

My parents hated Beckett, hated it when I started reading Beckett. 'You've been led astray by your brother!' they yelled. They hated Beckett's *nihilism*, his defeatism. 'And if I could begin it all over again,' Arsene goes on,

> knowing what I know now, the result would be the same. And if I could begin again a third time, knowing what I would know then, the result would be the same. And if I could begin it all over again a hundred times, knowing each time a little more than the time before, the result would always be the same, and the hundredth life as the first, and the hundred lives as one. A cat's flux.

A hundred lives as one. A cat's flux! I loved that. And now I discovered that it was the essence of Buddhism, and that I was supposed to be arriving at an awareness of this awfulness while meditating. So many people see reincarnation as reassuring, even wishful thinking – you don't die, you get another shot at it – but Beckett, like Buddha, knew better. Every existence plumps you right back on the rollercoaster of desire and disappointment, scratching yourself out of one itch into another. Best out of it! And too bad that suicide only thrusts you deeper into the *samsara* shit.

Nihilism was evil, my parents insisted. Just the way my mother said 'nihilism' gave it a dangerous foreign sound, like an Italian stiletto. Or like Nietzsche. Foreign names, evil foreign words. Nothing sensible and Anglo-Saxon about nihilism. Nihilism was of the devil, it was the beginning of all criminal behaviour. Who would ever behave if life was meaningless? Even worse, nihilism was the beginning of *not trying*, not making a wholesome Anglican effort to improve the world. God had created us in his image, life was good; if the Fall had left the world less than perfect, that was our fault and it was up to us to make it better. Not to bellyache. Nor to bail out like a wimp. Buddhist fatalism was evil and led people to corruption and despondency which was why millions were dying of hunger and disease in Asia. 'We know because we've been there,' my parents would say, referring to missionary trips to Malaysia, India, Pakistan.

All this when I was sixteen, seventeen.

Now, listening to the complacent, pessimistic Coleman, it occurred to me that Buddhism framed things differently. To perceive the emptiness at the heart of existence, you must *first* achieve purity. Far from being a plunge into criminal behaviour, such a vision was – how odd! – the *reward* for good behaviour, and a key in the first door that would get you out of gaol. It was impurities and ignorance that prevented you from seeing things as they really were (awful) and hence prompted you to grow attached to life and suffer. The person who perceives deeply that life is empty, must be morally admirable otherwise he could never have arrived at the concentration required to grasp this. Certainly, I thought, I had always had an impression of Beckett as somehow saintly, or at least hermit-like in his pessimism, hardly a man plagued by the desire for this world's goods.

On the other hand, and this was where it all grew complicated, there was no way I personally thought of life as a veil of misery. No way could I accept Coleman's vision. Or Beckett's, for that matter. Precisely the problem for me is that life is *so beautiful*. I am very attached to it. My misery when I was ill was only in part the pain. More important was losing beauty, being unable to enjoy. But I have never imagined joy was impossible.

Thus my confused reflections in the old monastery garden after that evening's talk, with the air now silvering to twilight and that grating music striking up in the valley below. It was beautiful being here, I decided, in this balmy air beneath the cypresses high on the Tuscan hills. The fairground noise had ceased to bother me. It was beautiful watching my fellow meditators cloaked in their thoughts at dusk, noble in their silence. There was a young woman, I remember, six or seven months pregnant, standing at the low parapet gazing down into the valley. Her fingers, just meeting on her belly, were relaxed and slender, and from time to time she turned her head this way and that, twisting her long neck, as if to relieve some stiffness there. Life is *too* beautiful, I decided. Not disgusting at all. There was a shadow of a smile on her lips. And the act of meditation was making it *more* beautiful, causing me to experience it more calmly. Simply eating had become an intense, slow pleasure, feeling a rough crust of bread on the roof of your mouth, a crisp carrot between your teeth, a forkful of rice melting in saliva on the tongue, slithering down the throat, then the cool cleanness of the water that washed it all away, the quiet sense of repletion. Sitting silently at table with the others was also an intense pleasure, watching their silent faces as they ate, watching their concentration. Breathing the evening air was beautiful.

I should definitely stop writing, I decided. How could I possess this deep calm day by day if I went on writing, hoping, fighting? I remembered Emil Cioran saying of Beckett that, if, over dinner, someone started discussing the relative merits of contemporary writers, Beckett would be furious and turn his chair to the wall in mute disgust. He

**I should definitely stop writing, I decided. How could I possess this deep calm day by day if I went on writing, hoping, fighting?**

refused to be part of such conversations. Wasn't all Beckett's later writing, it occurred to me, like Walser's tiny pencil script, an attempt to stop writing while still going on writing? First the switch to French – language, language, not *my* language – then the pieces getting shorter and shorter, with each sentence appearing to cancel out the one before, the whole thing more and more resistant to the reader, more and more concentrated on simple physical movements, walking, shifting the eyes, breathing. 'All writing is a sin against speechlessness,' Beckett had said. He would have stopped, I thought, if he could.

Again I recalled the evening I was at the Booker dinner. My acceptance speech churning in my head, I nevertheless prepared myself to clap when Arundhati Roy won. I think all of us on the shortlist knew that Arundhati Roy would win: the book was charming, it was already a bestseller, it was from India, it was about poor children who suffer abuse but make good, the author was beautiful without being too young, sophisticated without being a member of the English upper classes. How could she not win? I prepared myself to clap, and I *did* clap, damn it! And Arundhati Roy went to the podium and stood there smiling, beautifully – she was wearing a beautiful dress – and said she was lost for words, quite lost, because she had *never imagined* she could win, she hadn't prepared anything to say. And I knew this was false because I had been to lunch with her the day before and she seemed more than prepared to win. If nothing else, the bookmakers

were giving her as odds-on favourite. So this speech, like
the one I never delivered, had been carefully prepared, I
realised, and prepared, like mine, to seem modest and
unprepared, hence doubly false.

Then Salman Rushdie walked over to me and frowned
and said if it was him he would be furious; he would be
throwing chairs round and complaining that he should
have won. I smiled and said I *was* furious, but not in this
particular moment, just generally. Generally in a fury. If I
threw chairs around all the time there would be nowhere
for anyone to sit.

How can one lead such a life without running into an
ulcer or two?

Stop.

I suppose it has taken me an hour and more to write
down these last few reflections, but it only takes a second
or two for them to flash through the mind as you try to
focus on the breathing on your lips. How many times did
these ideas race through my head in the following days, in
the long silent dawns, in the guided sessions as Guru
Coleman invited us to explore our bodies, in the twilight
hour with the cackling nuns and the clashing music and
the strong cries of children playing outside the monastery
walls? Stop writing, I told myself. Enough. Enough.

Uncalled for, unwanted, the thoughts flew across my
mental space, back and forth, hither and thither, like birds
in the evening sky, chasing and losing and finding each
other, racing, wheeling, dispersing, gathering, gliding a

while then flapping in hard flight, always moving, through each other and across each other, at different altitudes, different speeds, as the light fails and the breeze comes up and the rain spatters on rustling leaves. Then one by one, at last, they begin to settle, they drop from view. With a last flutter, a thought settles on its perch and is quiet. On a rooftop perhaps, or in your wrist, in your throat. Another joins the first, and another. Thoughts fluffing their feathers before falling still. Perhaps one last squawk – *Rushdie was right! I should have hurled a chair!* – then silence. Until, huddled together on their wire, between your ears, they lose definition, merge into each other, become a single pool of feathery shadow, deep shadow in the darkness, one layer beneath another, beneath others, as eyes close behind closed eyelids, watched by still deeper eyes, and the mind at last discovers itself transparent.

It was on the sixth or seventh evening that I came to myself in the meditation room and found I was alone: the others had gone. I was late for bed.

# Coleman

ITCH BY ITCH, ache by ache, pulse by pulse, the body was explored. There was the first time I felt the roots of my teeth, a deep vibration in the gums, the first time the tongue throbbed and twitched and was truly present in my mouth, the first time a ball of fire rose slowly from stomach to chest. Pains flared, burned, petered out. Then returned.

Meantime one's personality was being stripped apart. It was a complicated demolition job where work had to proceed in a certain order: first this certainty came down, then that, then the one on the floor beneath. Not a sudden collapse but a steady dismantling. Or perhaps it was simply that without the people each side of you who make you who you are – wife, family, colleagues, friends – without work, TV, radio, without newspapers and books, phone and email, without a keyboard or paper to write on, the construct that was me was falling apart, rather as though a ship held together by the water it sailed in had been lifted into dry dock. Bits fell off. There was a day of tears, a day of confusion, a day of panic, a day of optimism.

'May all beings be free from all attachment,' Coleman intoned and he explained the pains we were experiencing thus: the body was an asbestos-clad stove full of burning coals. The coals were the smouldering accumulation of our past thoughts and actions. If we felt no heat in the ordinary way it was because the constant stimulation of our senses, the interminable churning of our mental activity, were powerful insulators: always moving, thinking, doing, we didn't notice. But by taking the five precepts and practising Anapana we had stripped off the asbestos and cracked open the stove. Then we felt our karma's painful heat. Now, day by day, with Vipassana, we would go into every corner of the stove, we would turn the coals so that they glowed and scorched. It was hard, he said. But slowly, surely, they would burn themselves out and all would be calm. Our minds would be pure and empty.

I thought: So they wait until the seventh day to tell you that the whole thing is based on pain, experiencing pain, accepting pain, something that, had you been informed beforehand, would most likely have deterred you from coming.

'Attachment to self,' Coleman said, 'is so strong that we will never be rid of it unless the suffering we feel within is stronger.' I remembered Beckett's *Endgame*. 'You must learn to suffer better than that, Clov, if you want them to weary of punishing you – one day.'

I had developed a curious state of mind during these evening talks. I believed nothing. I found the ideas ridiculous and contradictory: if life was utterly empty, how could you ascribe a value to purity, how could there be rules governing reincarnation based on your behaviour? etc, etc. At the same time I listened attentively, I enjoyed listening, and I saw that there were indeed ways in which Coleman's words could be applied to my experiences. I felt I knew what he meant when he spoke of everything flowing, mind and material dissolving into energy. Nor was it unthinkable that the strange pains I had been feeling had in some way to do with all those years sitting tensely, racking my brains over sheets of empty paper, building up hopes, rejoicing over some small achievement, over-reacting to setbacks and disappointments. And it was true that if you placed yourself, or your attention, as it were *beside* these pains, if you just sat together with them and let them be, not reacting or wishing them away, they did in the end subside. Likewise the thoughts: if you let them bubble up without judging them, or engaging them in any way, they gradually fizzled out. What's more, you felt that a certain serenity had been acquired in this process, an understanding that much of the pain we feel comes from our reaction to pain, much of our agitation from our excitement with agitation.

Above all, and more generally, I did sense the first hints of that famous equanimity Coleman was constantly speaking of. I had learned to put up with the lazy translation. I forgave our one-legged interpreter. In the end the guy seemed extremely pleasant, and now I was getting some perspective, not at all as incompetent as I had supposed. Some remarks he made in answer to people's questions were extremely helpful. I even forgave *myself* when, from time to time, I still grew irritated with him. Of the two, forgiving myself was harder. It came to me now that I'd always risen to the bait of yelling at myself, I'd always been determined to savour just how humiliating failure can be, and to make an exhibition of it. So this was progress, of a kind; paradoxically, letting go, you actually gained control, albeit of a different kind from the control you'd spent your life seeking. Distance, rather than grip. All you have to do now is stop writing, I decided, and you'll have clinched it. You'll have changed for ever.

But if I stopped writing, what would I do for a living? It was a false question. I had my teaching. I would be a teacher, a sort of servant. Robert Walser had been obsessed by the idea of service, of burying the ego in service. He dreamed of being a butler and actually worked as one for a while. I knew that this was a bridge too far for me. But teaching is an honest job. I enjoy teaching. With the writing behind me, the tussle in the mind would be over, likewise the gap between experience and fabricating a written account of experience, plus the foolish yearning for praise and success. All over. My health could only improve.

On the eighth morning I had an appointment to see Coleman. The afternoon check-ups had been suspended from day four. I wondered if this was because they were concerned that some of the more negative, aggressive participants might start a rebellion (one woman had used the word gulag when complaining about the rule against leaving the grounds); or because, with sixty people, they felt it was too much of a waste of time, too distracting to have everyone listen to everyone else. If you needed advice, they said, you could sign up for a fifteen-minute appointment with Coleman during the unguided meditation sessions on the seventh, eighth and ninth days.

My first thought was not to sign up. I had nothing to ask Coleman, or to tell him. If I wanted to know more about Buddhism, I could read about it, though I couldn't really see the point of pursuing notions so whimsical that I would never be able to accept them; those born in a rich, beautiful, peaceful country like Italy, Coleman had told us, could congratulate themselves on having scored highly in their previous lives. Ergo, those born in the Sudan had behaved badly. Nor did I imagine the guru would be interested in my views or reflections. Why should he be? Why should I want him to be? No, the only reason for my going to see Coleman would be curiosity, meaning, in my case, the possibility of collecting an interesting conversation to put in a book at some later date. Or in an article. I could write to the *New York Review* and ask them if they would be interested in an article on Vipassana meditation. Or to the *Guardian*.

But if you don't want to go on writing, what is the point of collecting things to write? Don't do it.

On the other hand, I *was* curious about Coleman. He was a type I'd never encountered before, a strange mix of blandness, serenity and shrewdness. He had spoken of an earlier life, in the 1950s and '60s, working for the CIA in Thailand before his search for a more tranquil state of mind led him to Burma, Buddhism and Vipassana. The anecdotes in his evening talks were infantile, deliberately so I had begun to sense, and delivered with a childish take-it-or-leave-it enthusiasm. He was deliberately insulting the intelligence, attempting to put that pesky faculty in its place. On the plus side, he had none of the sanctimoniousness that fatally attaches itself to every Christian clergyman. Nor did he wear any item of clothing that smacked of robe or ritual, or New Age vogue, for that matter. It was always: old slippers, shapeless pants, a colourless T-shirt. 'I had to have these pants made for me,' he announced apropos of nothing. 'Because I'm so fat.'

My immediate impression, then, was that the man was harmless. He wouldn't harm a fly, which was just as well, being a Buddhist. But once we shifted from the monotony of Anapana, to the more taxing adventure of Vipassana, I began to sense how powerful Coleman's charisma could be. He would wait until we were all settled in the meditation room before making his entrance. We would take off our shoes at the door, go to our places, reorganise our cushions, drag our ankles into place, arrange our hands in laps or on knees, close our eyes and settle. Only when we had been there for some minutes would we pick up the sound of slippers shuffling along the corridor. Outside, the guru would pause, as if he hadn't quite made up his mind whether to come in. Then the door clicked, creaked open, swung to and clicked shut again. Again he paused, standing at the threshold, and I remember having the impression that he liked to hold on to things for support, the door handle, the table where the translator sat. Or perhaps just to touch them. He liked to touch things. We listened to his footsteps, teasingly slow, as he made his way to his shabby armchair. He sighed heavily, slumped into the upholstery and was silent.

Behind our closed eyes, his presence filled the room, his laboured breathing became our breathing. The clock ticked. Sometimes, in the far distance, you might hear a train hooting, or, on one afternoon, very faintly, an ambulance. More often dogs barked, a chained dog barking at others passing by, I thought. Thoughts, thoughts. I made my objective note. The minutes passed. Coleman was silent. There was no hurry. At the same time a fine tension began to creep around the room, a collective waiting for his voice; when at last it did ring out, we started. It seemed to speak from inside us.

'May all beings live in peace.'

Guiding the meditations, Coleman had a deeper, more measured, sonorous voice than the one he used in his talks. 'May all beings be free from all attachment and all sorrow. May all beings be filled with happiness and sympathetic joy.'

'Sadhu Sadhu Sadhu.'

I didn't say the words myself, but I assented.

He began tamely. He had us focus on the breath for some minutes, the breath crossing the lip. When he didn't speak for a while, you wondered if he mightn't have fallen asleep. Then the voice boomed out again. No doubt because our eyes were closed and because we were sitting so still for so long, sounds became physical things. The clock ticked in fingers and toes. The gong that began and ended each session tingled in my cheeks. A door slamming was a slap. Coleman's voice clanged a bell in your chest. Your body rang.

'Now we will take our attention away from the breath,' he said calmly, 'and move it upwards to the top of the skull.' He began to lead us through our bodies, and when Coleman named a part of the body it really was easier for you to get in contact with it, easier than if you were meditating alone. Naming a part of the body, his voice touched it, but without using any mystical formulas. 'Now move your attention to your cheeks. To the left cheek. To the right cheek. To both cheeks. Pay attention. Take note of any sensation that arises in this part of the body.'

His timing was impressive. He would have you concentrate on a wrist, thigh, or shoulder to the point that it became an agony to be so focused. I had never imagined that this combination of emptying the mind of thought and concentrating it on physical sensation could be such hard work. 'Feel how the sensation changes, in your hands, the back of the hands, the fingers, the fingertips, constantly changes, infinitely nuanced, infinitely delicate; *anicca*, know *anicca*.'

Then after a long pause, just when it seemed you couldn't maintain this focus a moment longer, he would say: 'And now, let go. Not holding on to the sensation if it's pleasurable. Not fighting the sensation if it's painful. Just . . . let . . . go.'

And I did. It was as if Coleman, Coleman's voice, were able to command the same waves of release that had initially so surprised me when practising paradoxical relaxation. He commanded and I let go; a strange fluid rushed in, rigidity dissolved.

'Deeper,' Coleman insisted. 'Deeper and deeper, into the muscle, into the bone. Feel the sensation in the very bone. Feel that even the bone is subject to change. *Anicca*.'

We were concentrating on the arms, the elbows, and now it seemed I really was feeling the two bones in my right forearm. The ulna and the radius were present to me, their shape and consistency. It was the first time Coleman had invited us to go into the bone and, sceptical as I always am, I wondered if this was hypnotism. Was I the object of some clever hypnotic suggestion? But if it was hypnotism, would I be able to wonder if it was hypnotism?

'Let go,' Coleman said softly, 'just let go,' and another barrier went. I began to look forward to him saying the words. I was disappointed when he didn't. I realised that in the future, meditating alone at home, I would say this formula to myself – let go – imagining Coleman saying it, imagining his voice and the particular cadence he used, and I would feel how much more effective the words would have been if he were there in person to say them.

I decided I would, after all, make an appointment to see Coleman and signed myself in on the morning of the eighth day. Standing outside his door, I felt unexpectedly emotional. I had made a considerable effort over the last day or so not to plan a speech, or imagine the conversation, or even make a list of things to say. All the same, the meeting had begun to loom in my mind as something special. Outside his door I felt agitated. Something important was at stake. The feeling irritated me. I was an adult, canny, experienced and illusion-free. Why on earth was I going to talk to a guru?

With impressive punctuality, the woman before me came out of the room together with the translator and I went in and sat down. Coleman smiled and asked me if I had got my voice back and I said, 'Now we'll see.'

'Bravo!' he laughed.

It was a small sitting room with two armchairs arranged face to face and the shutters half closed against the August sun. I asked him how come he was limping so badly and he explained that they had been moving him around a conference complex in Malaysia on an open golf buggy when the driver braked hard and he had fallen out of the buggy and broken his hip.

Coleman spent some minutes describing the accident and the hospital. He seemed oddly enthusiastic about it all. 'The Malaysian nurses were wonderful!' Then he asked, 'But how are you getting on?'

I told him the retreat had stirred up a lot of emotions and reflections.

He waited.

I looked at him. He smiled at me. Not inviting, just waiting. The problem was, I said, that I didn't see how one could go on living the same way one always had and incorporate Vipassana into that. I felt this discipline was demanding pride of place, demanding that my whole life change.

Even as I said these portentous things I appreciated that had someone like myself made this kind of declaration, this admission of weakness, to my mother and father in their evangelical heyday, they would have had him on his knees giving his heart to Jesus in no time at all. There would have been tears and prayers and rivers of emotion. Coleman raised a bushy eyebrow. After a long pause he said: 'A lot of people get that idea into their heads.'

I was a little thrown. I waited but nothing more was forthcoming.

'Well,' I eventually said, 'I'm being asked to look on life as an affliction, a source of suffering, and to learn not to want it, whereas, the truth is I find the whole thing very beautiful. Living. These hills, the people here. I'm very attached to it all. Perhaps that's why I don't see how Vipassana is compatible. With the way I live, I mean. I keep feeling I'm being asked to say goodbye to life.'

Coleman was attentive, pleasant, distant. Again, after a pause, he said, 'Concentrate on *anicca*, get to know *anicca*.'

This did begin to sound like, 'Get to know our Lord

Jesus.' I felt annoyed. I could play mute as well as anyone, I decided. I wouldn't say anything else till he started taking the interview seriously.

We watched each other. He seemed to understand my decision and instead of prolonging the silence asked, 'What do you do for a living?'

'I teach translation. And write books.'

'How interesting. What kind of books?'

'Novels, essays.'

He sat smiling at me. I waited. Then I realised he was smiling because he knew I was waiting for him to ask another question about my books, so that I could talk about them. And he wasn't going to.

'I mean,' I said hurriedly, 'I wonder how one can square writing, desiring success, with Vipassana. I've been wondering if I should stop.'

'Vipassana?'

'No, writing.'

'Oh.' He frowned and sighed. 'You know, lots of people come to these retreats and get it into their heads they should retire to a monastery or something. I can't see why.'

I was beginning to find the encounter galling. 'Well, monks don't write books, do they? The two things are evidently incompatible.'

Again the slow smile. 'Monks don't do lots of things. Who said you have to be a monk?'

'The fact is, more than anything else, words seem to take me away from the present moment. I'm never really here. Always word-mongering. I feel a lot of what's wrong with my life comes from words.'

He always waited a while before replying.

'We're speaking now,' he eventually said. 'We're using words now. It's quite pleasant, isn't it? Maybe useful.'

'It's different with books.'

The way he watched made you feel that despite his eighty and more years, he was focused on you, he cared. Then the answers were offhand.

'But books are wonderful things.' He chuckled. 'I even wrote one myself way back.'

'*The Tranquil Mind.*'

'That's right.'

I had seen a copy on the table outside the meditation room.

'It's not a very good book, I don't think, but an effective way of communicating a lot of information to a large number of people.'

Realising I would get nowhere, I said abruptly, 'Mr Coleman, perhaps you could help me with a smaller thing. I have trouble sitting up straight when I'm meditating. Especially here. At home I seem to manage. Here my back just collapses. I keep feeling I'm going to keel over.'

Coleman reflected, or appeared to. Perhaps it was the merest performance.

'I used to have a lot of problems sitting up straight,' he said.

'But what can I do?'

He breathed deeply. 'I wonder why you want to sit up straight.'

'Well, because it would be more comfortable, for a start, better for my back. I'd breathe better.'

He seemed unconvinced. 'I wouldn't do anything about it.'

'It does seem a fair thing to want, though.'

He looked out of the window. Perhaps he was going senile. He was losing touch.

'Sure.' He turned back to me. 'Everybody would prefer to sit up straight, yes.' He waited. 'You know, sometimes, when things don't happen for us, it's because we want them too much.'

I was silent.

'*Anicca*,' he said. 'Concentrate on *anicca*.' He leaned forward and offered me his hand. 'It would be interesting to go on talking, but I only have fifteen minutes per person.'

So that was it! I shook his hand, smiled daggers and went to the door in a fury. I had demeaned myself coming to talk to a guru and he had barely acknowledged my existence. So much for acquiring wisdom. As I left, an elderly man was waiting to come in. Coleman was running to schedule.

I stood in the stone corridor. It had recently been renovated and whitewashed but the Gothic arches round the doorways still kept their antique feel. The window at the far end was a square of brilliant light around the dark candle of a cypress outside. I went to look. The hills were ablaze with dusty sunshine. Down on the lawn, smoking and sunning herself on a deckchair, was the pretty young woman I'd caught Coleman talking to the first days of the retreat. She was taking time out. Join her, I decided. The hell with it.

Downstairs, approaching the main entrance, I stopped. The old bastard had called my bluff. He had seen through me. I was that simple. I shook my head, hesitated, and turned back down the corridor.

I had never entered the meditation room in the middle of a session. I closed the door as quietly as I could, and even so, as it clicked, a tremor ran through the bodies around me. The door was at the back of the room where three or four people sat on chairs. I passed them and padded barefoot up the narrow space between the men, two by two on mats to the left, and the women, two by two to the right. The four windows along the right-hand wall were open and a soft summeriness drifted in. Nevertheless I was aware of an intense, still calm, a hum almost. There was a collective mental energy around me that seemed tangible, as though I were wading through a warm sea of mind.

Having reached my place, I stood still to take a last look. Rows and rows of seated and kneeling figures. A fat man on a mountain of cushions. A gaunt Arab-looking boy who used nothing more than a low block of wood for a seat. Some sat straight-backed, some bowed. There were smooth, untroubled faces, frowning faces, faces smiling

faintly. Some had all the gear, the oriental shawls, the cushions with esoteric symbols; some wore washed-out shorts,
shapeless T-shirts. The pregnant woman was serene in a
half lotus. One man rested his hands on his knees, the
palms turned up, forefinger and thumb just touching.
Another let his arms drop in his lap. Then I saw that the
elderly woman to my right had a fly on her cheek. A black
blowfly. It was walking up from her neck to her cheek. She
didn't flinch. The clock ticked. The fly followed her hair-
line above an ear. She had greying hair tied in a bun. Was
she aware of the creature or not?

I sat down. I was glad I had come back. I felt privileged
to have seen the room when everyone was so still and concentrated. I settled down as quietly as I could and closed
my eyes. My anger with Coleman had abated. He had been
right to suspect my reasons for wanting to sit up straight. I
wanted to prove I could do it, to myself and others. Exhibitionism. Perhaps he was right about the writing too.
Maybe the real change would be to stop trying to impress
myself with all this talk of drastic changes. 'A lot of people
get that idea into their heads,' he had said. And: 'I used to
have problems sitting up straight myself.' You and I are
alike and like the others too, he was saying. Don't look for
some special relationship with me because you're a tortured writer. He'd been very polite, I thought. He wasn't
proselytising, he wasn't out to recruit disciples. I closed
my eyes and waited for the breath to declare itself on my
upper lip.

# Charity

THINGS AS THEY ARE. This bowl. The table. White yoghurt. At the last breakfast I was overwhelmed by the sheer presence of it all. This bread, this square of butter. Things as they are. My hand. The blemished skin, a scarred knuckle, a dirty fingernail. Everything was intensely itself, source at once of fascination and indifference. Scattered crumbs, splashed milk. I gazed at them. As in a Cézanne, each object had been set free from the mesh of human interpretation. A cup beside a slice of melon. Absolutely themselves. I say the words now – cup, melon – but my mind at the time was wordless. The cup, the melon, were things without words, not in relation, not part of a sentence or a story. And there was no distance between us. I was in the cup, I was sticky with melon. Raising my eyes, I looked at the young man across the table, cheeks freshly shaven, a red T-shirt, a tattoo on his middle finger. The tattoo mimicked a ring, etched into his skin. I watched. He was holding a biscuit, using a knife to smear it with pink jam. It was too intense.

The jam was too pink. The strong fingers too present. I was touching them. The fingers were touching me. Watching was touching. Words protect us perhaps. Words keep the world at bay. I say that now. The thought didn't occur to me then. I was tongue-tied, there, in the middle of it all. I really was right there.

In slow motion we went to the meditation room. The man behind me took his place, eyes closed, lips pressed together. I hadn't heard him cough for days. The man in front was a sack of coal, bulk settling into bulk. The woman to my right perched electrically still; she was a bird, a parrot. She could fly off at any moment.

I closed my eyes and waited. Sure enough, other eyes opened in the dark. I was in the pitch dark putting out to sea. Mine was a frail craft, an oarless skiff. I wasn't concerned. I had put out to sea before without coming back. It wasn't a problem. The keel grated on the stones and bobbed free, free as the breath floating on my lip.

How quickly I'd got going!

Time passed. Despite sitting still, my body was twisting; my face had detached itself from my head, it was drifting away: lips, nose and eyes stretched and skewed like a gargoyle's. It didn't matter. The sea has its tides and currents. Looking across the space between skull and skin, I saw coils of grey smoke under my nostrils. I watched the smoke turn. It seemed extraordinarily delicate. The coils were very tight and fluffy among the hairs poking from my nostrils.

'May all beings,' Coleman's voice boomed out, 'be free from all attachment.' A tremor stiffened my back. I hadn't heard him come in. He sighed heavily and said, 'Today, our last day, the Metta bhavana. Today, the sharing of merits.' Raising his voice to its most vatic and hypnotic, Coleman began to read:

Though I speak with the tongues of men and of angels, and have not charity, I am become as sounding brass, or a tinkling cymbal.

Damn. The wave that swept across me now was the exact opposite of a wave of relaxation. Nothing could have jerked me more sharply out of my tranced focus on the present moment than these words, nothing could have thrust me more forcibly back into history and narrative. 1 Corinthians 13 was Dad's favourite passage from St Paul. For a moment my father's voice and Coleman's were one. My little boat sank like a stone.

And though I have the gift of prophecy, and understand all mysteries, and all knowledge; and though I have all faith, so that I could remove mountains, and have not charity, I am nothing.

Charity! My mind raced. Why was Coleman reading *this*? Did he know my past? I saw my father in the pulpit, robes gleaming in the sunlight that fell through the rose window on summer mornings, bald head gleaming. These were the words, he believed, that more than any other established Christianity's superiority. St Paul's great hymn to charity. Being read by a Buddhist.

And though I bestow all my goods to feed the poor, and though I give my body to be burned, and have not charity, it profiteth me nothing.

As Coleman read each verse so the one-legged translator read the Italian version. Knowing both languages, each blow struck twice.

*Se distribuissi anche tutti i miei beni ai poveri, e dessi il mio corpo ad essere bruciato, se non ho la carità, tutto questo non mi giova nulla.*

What did it mean 'though I give my body to be burned'? Why would anyone do that? I was right back in the world of words and angry questions, the world of my young self pitted against my dad's preaching, against every form of proselytising and coercion and mystery-mongering.

Charity suffereth long, and is kind; charity envieth not; charity vaunteth not itself, is not puffed up.

It was odd. I was furious with Coleman for reading this passage, for bringing back my father, my embattled adolescence, furious with him for ruining what I had supposed would be another long, peaceful emptying of the mind into the spell of the present. At the same time, how could I not assent to these words? How could I not see that they were in line with all I had been thinking? Charity vaunteth not itself. It is not forever preparing prize acceptance speeches. Ergo, self-regard is uncharitable. How right that was! And though I sell a billion copies of my next novel, though I win the Nobel twice over and join the holy canon of literary greats, and have not charity, I am nothing.

Charity doth not behave itself unseemly, seeketh not her own, is not easily provoked, thinketh no evil; rejoiceth not in iniquity, but rejoiceth in the truth; beareth all things, believeth all things, hopeth all things, endureth all things.

This was mad. How can you believe all things, hope all things? For some reason I was on the brink of tears. I tried to remember a sermon where my father had explained the different words for love in the Bible, told his congregation why the word here had been translated as charity rather than love. I couldn't. I couldn't recall it. I must swallow down these emotions. The storm had blown up so quickly. There had been no warning.

Charity never faileth: but whether there be prophecies, they shall fail; whether there be tongues, they shall cease; whether there be knowledge, it shall vanish away.

Right, all this was so right! Whether there be novels, they shall disappear from the shelves. Only a month after publication most likely. And essays and articles and newspapers and websites and even the most beautiful poems. Though your book last a thousand years, though it last a hundred thousand, it will vanish. You are nothing.

But wouldn't charity vanish too? a cool voice remarked. What did it mean, charity never faileth? That was empty piety.

For we know in part, and we prophesy in part. But when that which is perfect is come, then that which is in part shall be done away.

Listening to Coleman's deep voice, listening to the translator's lame echo, I realised I had never really taken in this passage before. It had always been one of those irritating parts of the Bible that obliged you to acknowledge that Christianity wasn't all silly, that St Paul wasn't just an anal retentive. Here we know 'in part'. That was exactly the problem. Knowledge comes in parts. The urologist, the neurologist, the psychologist. And the mathematician, the linguist, the climatologist. Even in daily conversation, every word divides the world in parts. But when that which is perfect is come . . .

What? What is perfect? And when?

I opened my eyes and watched Coleman read. Like my father, he knew the text so well he barely needed to look at it.

When I was a child, I spake as a child, I understood as a child, I thought as a child: but when I became a man, I put away childish things. For now we see through a glass, darkly; but then face to face: now I know in part; but then shall I know even as also I am known.

Did I ever become a man? I wondered. And what would it mean, to know as one was known? Who really knows me anyway? Nobody. Despite all your novels and half confessions, nobody knows you. There was something very fine about the words 'through a glass darkly', so fine that you hardly wanted to know things any other way. Through a glass darkly was OK by me.

Coleman paused and launched into the last great verse:

For now abideth faith, hope, charity, these three; but the greatest of these is charity.

Why, I demanded – my head shaking slowly from side to side – why why why wasn't it possible for me to have the benefits I had no doubt obtained from this retreat, from this meditative practice, the mindful breathing, the exploration of the body, the growing awareness and equanimity, without bringing in these religious imponderables that always shake me up so badly? Why couldn't Coleman have done one last session of Vipassana and sent us off happily home?

The guru was talking now. By the end of our ten-day retreat, he was saying, we should have reached the stage known as *sotapanna*, 'he who has entered the stream', sometimes also called *sotapatti*, 'stream-winner'. He smiled blandly. He hoped it would be clear how these words related to the discipline we had been following. We had been learning to enter the stream. *Anicca*. But we hadn't done this exclusively for our own benefit. We weren't here to gaze at our navels. The very hard work we had done, he said, had accumulated for each of us a large number of merits. Every moment's escape from the confines of our narrow egos was transformed into a wealth of merits. Now, if we shared these merits with others, we could help them, we could improve the world.

How beautiful St Paul was, I thought. At least in that one passage on charity. At least in the King James version. And what drivel Coleman was talking.

There followed one of those strange half-hours where the intellect is hopelessly at war with the emotions. Our guru rambled on about merits and how, by sharing them with others, they actually multiplied for you too, so the more you shared your merits the more merits you had to share. We would embark now, he said, on the Metta bhavana, or meditation of loving kindness, which involved thinking intensely first of those closest to us, wishing them well, then the wider family, then, gradually, those we knew less well, those we didn't know at all, those who suffered in every corner of the globe, and those who killed and tortured and raped, even those who pushed destruction's buttons in the Pentagon, the Kremlin. We would share our merits with them and improve their lives and ours.

Crap. If one could save the world thinking good thoughts, it would have been done time ago.

While Coleman spoke, people fidgeted, nodding their heads, or shaking them, swaying from side to side, shifting their weight here and there. It was interesting that the moment you lost the concentration of Anapana and Vipassana it became impossible to maintain the meditation position. You had to move. I wondered if the others felt as embarrassed as I did by all this.

Coleman invited us to think of our parents. We were to close our eyes again, to concentrate on our parents, to recall their faces, to recall all they had done for us, to share our merits with our father and mother, to wish them well. 'May they be free from all attachment. May their lives be full of happiness and sympathetic joy. I gladly share all my merits with them.'

I thought of my dead father, my ageing, sick, but still sprightly mother. Naturally I couldn't wish my father well, because he was dead.

Could I?

**Crap. If one could save the world thinking good thoughts, it would have been done time ago**

Or could I?

I mean logically I couldn't, but what if I did wish him well anyway? What harm could it do for me to wish my father well? It was meaningless because Dad was beyond harm and beyond being well. He was beyond being. On the other hand, it couldn't harm, could it, for Christ's sake? Is it such a problem to do something meaningless?

Why was this bothering me so much?

I wished my mother well.

Wish your father well, a voice said. I resisted. It makes no fucking sense to wish my father well. He's dead. I won't have anything to do with this mumbo-jumbo and he wouldn't want me to, or rather, wouldn't have wanted me to. In fact, he would have been the first person to tell me to get up and walk out of this pagan bullshit right away. I smiled. Anglican through and through, Dad loathed the Catholic practice of praying for the dead. 'Paganism!' he would shake his head. 'Sheer, unadulterated paganism!' If I couldn't remember his face clearly, I had his voice spot on.

I wish my mother well because I always wish my mother well. I won't share my merits with her because I can't possibly believe in the claptrap of metaphysical accountancy. Next we'll be selling indulgences. Next we'll be lighting candles by photos of the dear departed.

Jesus!

I was stuck. Why? Why was all this emotional stuff happening? Why couldn't I just have sorted out my bellyaches and peeing problems and got right back to work?

I wish my father well, I thought.

How strange it seemed to say those words in my head! Dad has been dead so long. We argued before he died. I wish him well. We argued because I would not say, standing beside his bed, his deathbed, I would not say that I believed in God, that I was a Christian, to please him. 'I'm sure you do believe, Timothy,' he said. His face was grey, spectral. 'Tell me you do.' His lips barely moved. It was two days before he died. He stank. 'No.' I stood my ground. I wouldn't say the words for him because they weren't true. I wasn't a Christian. 'You shouldn't ask me to say such things.' I had been furious. It was the most underhand coercion.

Dad, I wish you well.

Then I sensed a stirring of the mind, a deep well-wishing in the mind, in the belly, in the bowels, that wasn't the words I was rehearsing, but that had been awakened or revealed by those words. Light had fallen on a dark place. I really did wish my father well, *enormously*. I was *bursting* with well-wishing for my father. There was a rolling ocean of well-wishing in me. Where had it come from?

'Maybe we have issues with those close to us. They have made us suffer. How we have suffered for the way they have behaved! And we have made them suffer. No doubt they too have suffered a great deal.' Coleman paused and sighed. 'All the same, I willingly share my merits with them. I share my merits with them gladly. May their lives be full of happiness and sympathetic joy.'

It was really too bad I couldn't believe in this merits claptrap. There was such a deep ring of sincerity in Coleman's voice. I began to have a little respect for him, even though it was intellectually disqualifying to hold such nutty points of view. I fell to thinking of my wife. How we had made each other suffer!

Don't go there.

Our children. Our three children. My brother. My sister.

Faces appeared. I remembered those moments on the terrace at Maroggia. It was the same story, more controlled now, but the same. Something in this business of sitting still, emptying the mind of self-regard, settling into your flesh and blood, something in the soft breathing and the long hours just being there, just accepting that you really were here, here today and gone tomorrow that is; at some point it opened your heart.

There. I have used words that normally make me cringe. It opened your heart to the people around you. Suddenly you wished them well. Even people you really did not wish well. Now you did. However briefly. It brought down barriers and blurred boundaries. In your muscles, first, and your mind. Inside you. Rigidities, routines. They broke down. The mind melted in the flesh. The gap between you and the breakfast utensils shrank, between you and the landscape, between you and the people sitting beside you. We were all on a level. On the eighth or ninth day I had found myself sitting on a bench in the garden, a cup of herb tea in my hand, when the man who had talked about shaving his moustache to feel the breath on his lip came and sat down beside me. It was the only bench in the shade. He was a big athletic man in his early forties, I suppose. The sun was hot. We were sitting a foot or two apart, on the bench, and did not look at each other. We observed the Noble Silence. Yet at once there was an uncanny communion between us. I felt it instantly, intensely, and I knew he was feeling it too. We both knew, without having looked for it or wanted it, that the other was feeling a deep sympathy, a knowledge, but devoid of content. A knowledge of each other. We were both surprised and knew we were surprised. We were both glad, quietly. It must have lasted some minutes. I didn't know him from Adam.

Was this charity?

How can you, I wondered, as Coleman shared his merits now with American generals and Iraqi suicide bombers, how can you pretend to escape from the compartmentalisation of Western medicine and then complain when people go the whole hog and talk spirituality and aura and reincarnation?

How can you? Where draw the line?

Believeth all things. Hopeth all things.

Perhaps it's impossible to integrate mind and body without integrating both with everything.

Would it have been charity to tell my father I believed in God, even if I didn't? I don't.

Suffereth long, and is kind.

I wish you well, Dad.

I couldn't listen to Coleman. 'How they must suffer for

their crimes,' he was saying of Bush and Blair and Putin and bin Laden. 'I gladly share all my merits with them.' Coleman was mad. I went back to St Paul, to Dad's first love. If I have all those wonderful skills, he says, which are just a part, or parts, and have not charity, then I am nothing. It profiteth nothing. Because incomplete, transitory. The part is nothing. Charity is beyond parts, beyond boundaries, beyond time. Hence beyond words. Defined by negatives. It vaunteth not. It faileth not. Or by the absence of exclusions. Beareth believeth hopeth endureth all things. Perhaps it was charity, then, that I had been learning through Vipassana. The knowledge that you are one with the whole. Perhaps the day will come, I thought, when the water snakes rise beside my little boat and I will bless them with all my heart.

'Your vow of silence is lifted,' Coleman said. 'You may talk.'

At once there was movement in the meditation room, there was noise, commotion. I was astonished how eager everyone was to speak, to know each other, how loudly they cried out their names. People jumped from their mats and were shaking hands, saying hello, introducing themselves. Shrill voices, deep voices. Eye contact, gestures, multiplicity. A camera flashed.

In a daze I had just reached the door when a young woman danced up to me, barefoot, beaming.

'Are you, by any chance,' this pretty woman asked, 'Tim Parks, the writer?'

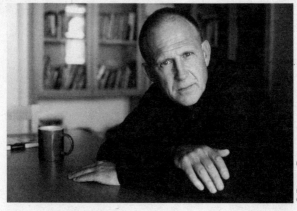

© Basso Cannarsa

TIM PARKS is an author, translator, critic and teacher. Born in Manchester to deeply religious parents, he grew up in London and studied at Cambridge and Harvard before moving to Italy where he has lived ever since.

He is the author of fourteen novels which have brought him the Somerset Maugham, Llewellyn Rhys and Betty Trask awards and a shortlisting for the Booker Prize. He has also written non-fiction about Italy, football, reading, translation, the Medicis and trains. His one hobby is white-water kayaking, which he hopes to pursue into extreme old age.

Tim Parks now meditates every day and claims to have remained absolutely calm the mornings after both the Brexit referendum and the election of Donald Trump.

RECOMMENDED BOOKS BY TIM PARKS:

*Teach Us to Sit Still*
*Europa*
*Italian Ways*
*Where I'm Reading From*

# How do we find Calm in our modern world?

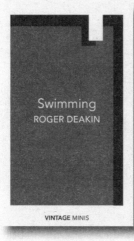

Swimming
ROGER DEAKIN

VINTAGE MINIS

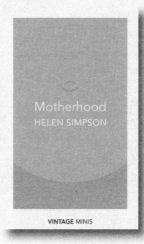

Motherhood
HELEN SIMPSON

VINTAGE MINIS

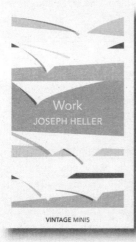

Work
JOSEPH HELLER

VINTAGE MINIS

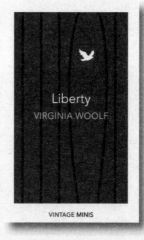

Liberty
VIRGINIA WOOLF

VINTAGE MINIS

## VINTAGE MINIS

The Vintage Minis bring you the world's greatest writers on the
experiences that make us human. These stylish, entertaining little
books explore the whole spectrum of life – from birth to death,
and everything in between. Which means there's something
here for everyone, whatever your story.